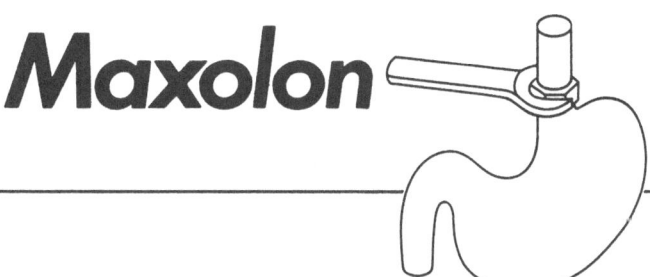

To Sue and Jenny
and our children

# MANAGEMENT OF COMMON DISEASES IN FAMILY PRACTICE

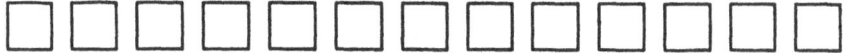

Series Editors: J. Fry and M. Lancaster-Smith

# GASTROENTEROLOGY

**M. Lancaster-Smith,** BSc, MD, FRCP

*Consultant Physician, Queen Mary's Hospital,
Sidcup, Kent*

and

**C. Chapman,** BSc, MB, BS, MRCS, LRCP

*General Practitioner, Maldon, Essex*

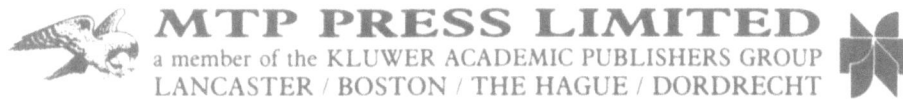

**MTP PRESS LIMITED**
a member of the KLUWER ACADEMIC PUBLISHERS GROUP
LANCASTER / BOSTON / THE HAGUE / DORDRECHT

Published in the UK and Europe by
MTP Press Limited
Falcon House
Lancaster, England

British Library Cataloguing in Publication Data

Lancaster-Smith, Michael
    Gastroenterology. — (Management of common
    diseases in family practice)
    1.  Gastrointestinal system — Diseases
    I.  Title        II  Chapman, C,        III.  Series
    616.3'3       RC801

ISBN-13: 978-94-011-7783-2          e-ISBN-13: 978-94-011-7781-8
DOI: 10.1007/978-94-011-7781-8

Typeset by UPS Blackburn, 76-80 Northgate, Blackburn, Lancashire.

# Contents

Series Editors' Foreword     vii

Introduction     ix

Acknowledgements     x

1. Gastro-oesophageal Reflux     1

2. Dysphagia     9

3. Nausea and Vomiting     19

4. Uncomplicated Peptic Ulcer     25

5. Complicated Peptic Ulcer     39

6. Surgical Management of Peptic Ulcer     45

7. Gastrointestinal Bleeding     57

8. Acute Abdominal Pain     65

9. Chronic Abdominal Pain     75

10. Acute Diarrhoea     83

11.  Chronic Diarrhoea                                          93

12.  Malabsorption                                              101

13.  The Irritable Bowel Syndrome                               111

14.  Ulcerative Proctocolitis and Crohn's Disease              117

15.  Diverticular Disease of the Colon                          129

16.  Constipation and other Problems with Defaecation          133

17.  Miscellaneous Gastrointestinal Problems                   141

18.  Jaundice and Common Liver Diseases                        145

     Appendix: Patient Information Sheets and Diets            165

     Bibliography                                              183

     Index                                                     187

# Series Editors' Foreword

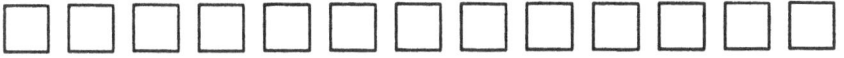

Effective management logically follows accurate diagnosis. Such logic often is difficult to apply in practice. Absolute diagnostic accuracy may not be possible, particularly in the field of primary care, when management has to be on analysis of symptoms and on knowledge of the individual patient and family.

This series follows that on *Problems in Practice* which was concerned more with diagnosis in the widest sense and this series deals more definitively with general care and specific treatment of symptoms and diseases.

Good management must include knowledge of the nature, course and outcome of the conditions, as well as prominent clinical features and assessment and investigations, but the emphasis is on what to do best for the patient.

Family medical practitioners have particular difficulties and advantages in their work. Because they often work in professional isolation in the community and deal with relatively small numbers of near-normal patients their experience with the more serious and more rare conditions is restricted. They find it difficult to remain up-to-date with medical advances and even more difficult to decide on the suitability and application of new and relatively untried methods compared with those that are 'old' and well proven.

Their advantages are that because of long-term continuous care for their patients they have come to know them and their families well and are able to become familiar with the more common and less serious diseases of their communities.

This series aims to correct these disadvantages by providing practical information and advice on the less common, potentially serious conditions, but at the same time to talk note of the special features of general medical practice.

To achieve these objectives, the *titles* are intentionally those of accepted body systems and population groups.

The *co-authors* are a specialist and a family practitioner so that each can supplement and complement the other.

The *experience bases* are those of the district general hospital and family practice. It is here that the day-to-day problems arise.

The *advice and presentation* are practical and have come from many years of conjoint experience of family and hospital practice.

The *series* is intended for family practitioners – the young and the less than young. All should benefit and profit from comparing the views of the authors with their own. Many will coincide, some will be accepted as new, useful and worthy of application and others may not be acceptable, but nevertheless will stimulate thought and enquiry.

Since medical care in the community and in hospitals involves teamwork, this series also should be of relevance to nurses and others involved in personal and family care.

JOHN FRY
M. LANCASTER-SMITH

# Introduction

Our purpose in this book is to provide a guide for general practitioners who are frequently faced with problems related to the digestive system, rather than a comprehensive text book of gastroenterology.

Emphasis has been placed on, and the majority of space devoted to, problems and diseases with which patients commonly present to the surgery. Many can be managed readily in general practice following minimal investigation. Others may require hospital referral for diagnosis and treatment. Nevertheless, even in this category of gastrointestinal disease, many are recurrent or chronic disorders and it is therefore inevitable that the general practitioner will have an important role in the long term management of such conditions.

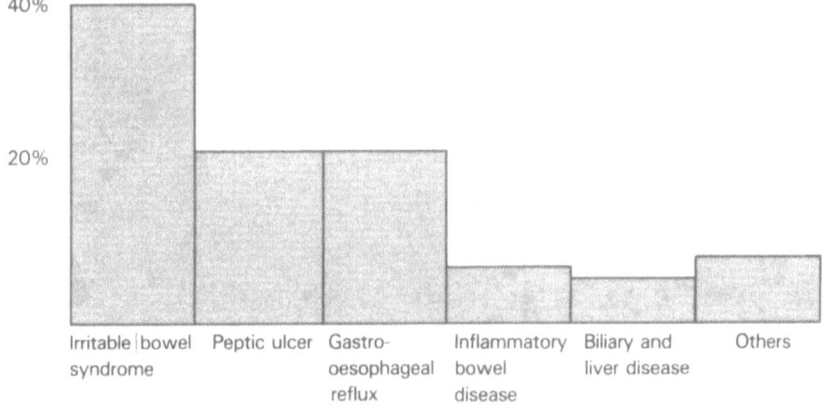

**Figure** New referrals to Gastrointestinal Clinic, Queen Mary's Hospital, Sidcup, Kent, 1983

For much of the book we have adopted a problem-orientated approach with chapters covering abdominal pain, diarrhoea, constipation, nausea, vomiting, dysphagia, malabsorption, jaundice and gastrointestinal haemorrhage. By contrast, chapters are devoted to specific common alimentary tract diseases including, gastro-oesophageal reflux, peptic ulcer, inflammatory bowel disease, the irritable bowel syndrome and diverticular disease.

# Acknowledgements

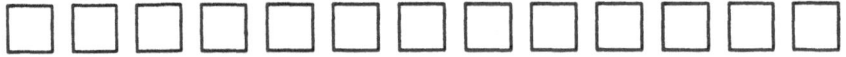

We wish to thank Miss Liz Valori and the Dietetic Department of Queen Mary's Hospital, Sidcup for allowing us to publish the diets included in the Appendix. We are also extremely grateful to Mrs Karen Brickenden and Mrs Amanda Lewer for preparing the final manuscript.

# 1

# Gastro-oesophageal Reflux

Gastro-oesophageal reflux is the commonest disorder of the oesophagus and accounts for approximately 20% of referrals to a district general hospital gastrointestinal clinic.

## ANTIREFLUX MECHANISMS

The *lower oesophageal sphincter*, which is formed by 4 cm of distal oesophageal circular smooth muscle, is the most important antireflux device. After relaxing to allow liquids or solids to enter the stomach it rapidly regains its tone, thus preventing reflux of gastric contents. It is also able to increase its tone still more in response to rises in intragastric and intra-abdominal pressures. The other antireflux mechanisms are illustrated in Figure 1.1. The so-called pinchcock action of the diaphragm probably plays only a small part but the intra-abdominal segment of the oesophagus below the diaphragm which acts as a flap valve is much more important. Any rise in abdominal pressure which raises intragastric pressure and encourages reflux will also squeeze equally upon the intra-abdominal oesophagus, thus helping to suppress reflux. Despite these mechanisms most of us intermittently reflux small amounts of gastric fluid due to transient relaxation of the lower oesophageal sphincter. This is rapidly returned to the stomach by reflex muscle action of the distal oesophagus, so-called *secondary peristalsis*.

Symptoms and pathological changes occur when the oesophageal mucosa has excessive contact with gastric contents as a consequence of continual or recurrent failure of the antireflux mechanisms. Faulty gastric emptying is an·

additional reason for increased reflux of gastric contents into the distal oesophagus.

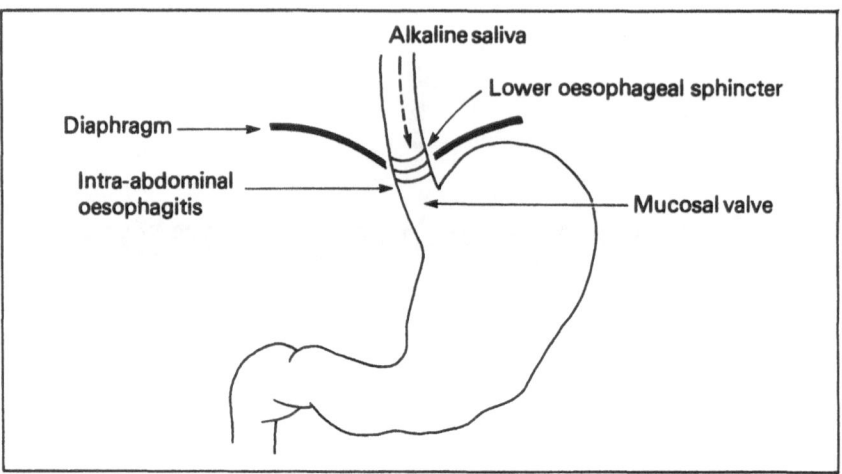

**Figure 1.1** Anti-gastroesophageal reflux mechanisms (from Lancaster-Smith, M. and Williams, K. (1982) *Problems in Gastroenterology*. (Lancaster: MTP Press))

## CONTROL OF MUSCLE ACTIVITY

The control of this motor activity is not entirely clear but it is known that an intact myenteric plexus of the oesophageal wall is essential for organized peristalsis. Parasympathetic activity and cholinergic transmitters increase and stimulation by the sympathetic nervous system and adrenergic transmitters decrease tone in the lower oesophageal sphincter. In addition to nervous control, hormones from the upper gastrointestinal tract also affect lower oesophageal function. Although their exact roles are not yet fully understood, gastrin increases lower oesophageal sphincter tone, whereas secretin has the opposite effect.

## HEARTBURN

Heartburn is the characteristic symptom of gastro-oesophageal reflux and is due to irritation of the oesophageal mucosa. The pain probably arises directly from nerve endings in this hypersensitive mucosa whenever there is persistent exposure to irritants such as hydrochloric acid and bile from the stomach. The same pain occurs when hot drinks or alcoholic spirits come into contact with reflux damaged mucosa. Although in some instances hypersensitivity progresses to frank oesophagitis, inflammatory changes are not present in all patients with heartburn. Why pain arises from the mucosa in the absence of inflammation is not clear but presumably constant contact with noxious substances renders the mucosa more permeable to irritants and the nerve endings more sensitive. It also seems likely that at least some pain results from *spasm in the muscle of the distal oesophagus*.

Heartburn, as with other sensations from the oesophagus, is usually felt retrosternally but may also be felt high in the epigastrium and along the costal margins. Radiation to the back of the thorax, neck, shoulders, arms and even the ears is not uncommon.

As the name implies, patients frequently describe the pain as burning which is felt particularly soon after a meal or whilst swallowing hot liquids or alcoholic spirits. On other occasions the pain will be likened to a lump stuck in the chest or throat. This sensation is possibly due to spasm of distal oesophageal muscle. In contrast to true dysphagia this sensation comes on after a meal and not whilst eating and there is no actual hold-up of food.

There are a number of other helpful pointers to pain suspected of being due to gastro-oesophageal reflux. Regurgitation of acid or bitter gastric contents into the mouth often occurs. Both regurgitation and heartburn may be brought on by bending or lying down. Antacids or belching often give relief.

## BLEEDING

Blood loss from oesophagitis may be a rare presentation of gastro-oesophageal reflux. This may be acute and result in haematemesis or melaena, or occult leading to symptoms of anaemia.

## ASPIRATION

Gastric contents may occasionally reach the pharynx when aspiration into the lungs can occur. This is particularly likely when recumbent, and gastro-oesophageal reflux should be considered in all patients with nocturnal wheezing or coughing.

## MANAGEMENT

### Diagnosis

*When these symptoms occur together there is no diagnostic problem and investigation is unnecessary.*

3

Unfortunately the situation is not always so clear cut and the diagnosis may have to be distinguished from other oesophageal diseases, peptic ulcer and gallbladder disease.

In addition, because of its site and radiation heartburn can also be confused with the pain of myocardial ischaemia. However, cardiac pain is usually more severe and described as gripping or crushing and not burning. It is frequently brought on by exertion and not by stooping or lying. There is often accompanying dyspnoea and not belching or regurgitation. The problem can sometimes be further resolved by the therapeutic test of asking the patient to note whether glyceryl trinitrate or antacids give the greater relief.

Nevertheless, there will be a small number in whom the diagnosis is not clear. Both these and those who fail to respond adequately to therapy will require further investigation.

## Barium meal

Barium studies have two main purposes. One is to exclude other disorders of the gastrointestinal tract, such as peptic ulcer or carcinoma of the gastric cardia in which reflux symptoms may be prominent. The second is to demonstrate that reflux will occur and whether there is an accompanying *sliding hiatus hernia*, which predisposes to reflux because the intra-abdominal segment of oesophagus is lost. Nevertheless, it is important to realize that failure to show a hernia does not exclude the diagnosis of gastro-oesophageal reflux as this can certainly exist in those without a hiatus hernia. It should also be stressed that a hernia itself does not cause symptoms unless accompanied by reflux. Likewise, some patients only have intermittent reflux and the radiologist may not be able to confirm its presence despite using various manoeuvres to stress the antireflux mechanisms.

## Endoscopy

Examination of the oesophagus, stomach and proximal duodenum with a flexible fibreoptic endoscope is a safe and well tolerated outpatient procedure now available in most district general hospitals. Obvious inflammatory changes of *oesophagitis* assessed either by direct vision or histologically may not always be present even in patients with severe heartburn. Thus, to some extent endoscopy has proved disappointing in the investigation of gastro-oesophageal reflux. Nevertheless, it may be helpful when diagnosis or management is proving difficult and is obligatory if, in addition to heartburn, there is dysphagia, anorexia, weight loss or vomiting.

4

## Acid perfusion test

If there is still doubt about the diagnosis of heartburn its precipitation by the perfusion into the distal oesophagus of N/10 hydrochloric acid and subsequent relief with sodium bicarbonate may be helpful.

## Manometry

In rare cases more information about the competence of the lower oesophageal sphincter can be obtained by intraluminal pressure measurements.

## Objective measurement of reflux episodes

Intraluminal pH probes and scintiscanning can be used to record the frequency of reflux and duration that gastric contents remain in contact with oesophageal mucosa due to defective secondary peristalsis. *Such procedures are only indicated when the other simpler and more readily available techniques have failed to confirm the diagnosis.*

## Treatment

The management of most cases of heartburn poses few problems. The aims of treatment can be considered under the following headings.

### Improve antireflux mechanisms

The first aim is to *improve the efficiency of the antireflux mechanisms and reduce the demands made upon them*. Certain foods, particularly *fats*, regularly cause heartburn and probably do so by changing the levels of the hormones that control lower oesophageal sphincter tone. The patient has usually discovered this for himself and taken the necessary action. *Alcohol* and *smoking* both reduce the efficiency of the lower oesophageal sphincter and should be avoided, especially at meal times. *Metoclopramide* (Maxolon and Primperan), as it improves lower oesophageal sphincter function, enhances secondary peristalsis and speeds gastric emptying, is worthy of trial. It should be taken prior to meals and before going to bed.

### Reduce intragastric pressure

Warning should be given not to take large meals and large volumes of fluid or to drink with a meal as this may increase intragastric pressure to a level that overcomes the antireflux mechanisms. This is most likely to happen when the meal is followed by lying down, slumping in a chair or stooping. Specific advice must therefore be given about posture even to the extent of raising the head of the bed by about 10 cm or elevating the mattress with pillows beneath the head end.

*Reduction of weight* is a great help when the patient is overweight, even if only a few kilograms are shed. This results in a lowering of intra-abdominal pressure but the benefit is probably as much due to the accompanying reduction in size of meals.

Tight garments such as girdles and long-line bras should not be worn.

### Reduction of gastric acidity

Pain from a hypersensitive or inflamed mucosa will be decreased by *making gastric contents less acidic*. This can be achieved by regular therapy over a period of a few weeks rather than just when symptoms arise. Taken at this frequency it is probably best to use a combined aluminium and magnesium preparation to avoid bowel disturbance.

Antacids, in addition to their local intraluminal action, tend to reduce reflux itself because alkalinization of the stomach contents increases lower oesophageal sphincter tone.

The $H_2$-antagonists cimetidine (Tagamet) and ranitidine (Zantac), by suppressing gastric acid secretion will even more predictably reduce acidity.

Preparations combining antacids with polysiloxanes (Asilone, Andursil, Polycrol) are said to form a protective layer and by dispersing intragastric gases reduce belching and reflux. Alginates (Gaviscon, Gastrocote) from an alkaline 'raft' on the gastric contents which suppresses reflux and prevents contact of the gastric fluid and oesophageal mucosa.

### Pyrogastrone

Liquorice extracts enhance healing of gastric and duodenal ulcers. Their action depends upon contact with the mucosal surface (see Chapter 4). A new product, Pyrogastrone, which combines alginate and carbenoxolone, is intended to deliver the active substance to the inflamed oesophageal mucosa and promote healing.

When spasm of the oesophagus appears to be the major component of pain, sublingual *trinitrine* should be tried.

*It should again be stressed that regular antacids prove successful in the great majority of patients with heartburn and other products are only necessary when these have failed.*

Drugs such as atropine, hyoscine, belladonna and synthetic 'antispasmodics' reduce tone in the lower oesophageal sphincter and are, therefore, contraindicated in heartburn.

## Longterm management

Patients should be warned that as with other peptic disorders recurrence is common. They should be instructed to recommence treatment at the first suggestion of an exacerbation and constantly reminded about the general measures that reduce the incidence of reflux.

Long remissions from symptoms are usual and this is probably due to the fact that lower oesophageal sphincter tone and secondary peristalsis improve with healing of the mucosal lesion, thus breaking the vicious circle.

Patients should be instructed to reattend the surgery if the usual symptoms change, especially if food begins to stick during swallowing.

## Special problems

Apart from hiatus hernia and obesity, which have already been mentioned, there are two other common situations which predispose to gastro-oesophageal reflux, pregnancy and gastric surgery.

*Pregnancy* is often accompanied by heartburn and is probably encouraged by a rise in intra-abdominal pressure and a reduction in the tone of the lower oesophageal sphincter.

Patients who have undergone *gastric surgery*, including vagotomy, are prone to heartburn. This is partly caused by irritant bile salts which frequently reflux into the stomach following such operations. In addition vagotomy renders the lower oesophageal sphincter incapable of increasing tone in response to a rise of intragastric pressure. Aluminium hydroxide or hydrotalcite (Altacite), both of which bind bile salts, should therefore be taken regularly until symptoms are relieved.

A fortunately much rarer condition that also predisposes to gastro-oesophageal reflux is *scleroderma*. This is because involvement of the oesophageal muscle leads to impaired peristalsis and inefficient clearing of the gullet. The lower oesophageal sphincter is also commonly affected, which allows free flow of gastric contents into the oesophagus. In addition to the symptoms of heartburn and regurgitation, true dysphagia can occur either from impaired peristalsis or from peptic stricture. All that can be offered are those measures prescribed for other severe cases of gastro-oesophageal reflux.

## Referral for surgery

*Only a very small number of patients with heartburn will require surgery* and in these cases there is frequently a substantial coexisting hiatus hernia. The operations with the greatest chance of success aim to reduce the hernia and establish an intra-abdominal segment of oesophagus. The indications for referral to the surgeons are: (1) failure of enthusiastic and compliant medical treatment to relieve symptoms or heal oesophagitis; (2) recurrent haemorrhage either from oesophagitis or an actual oesophageal ulcer – this may present as haematemesis or melaena requiring admission to hospital – however, it is usually occult and *all patients with recurrent heartburn should have a haemoglobin estimation as chronic blood loss and anaemia frequently go undetected both by patient and doctor*; and (3) stricture which results from chronic oesophagitis and leads to dysphagia (see Chapter 2).

---

- The great majority of patients with uncomplicated gastro-oesophageal reflux will respond to adequate antacid therapy and where appropriate weight reduction.

- When these measures fail other preparations, such as cimetidine, metoclopramide, Pyrogastrone, Gaviscon or Gastrocote should be tried.

- Check haemoglobin concentration as anaemia may go unnoticed.

- Other investigations are only necessary when diagnosis is unclear or when there is accompanying *dysphagia* or *anorexia*.

- The demonstration of an hiatus hernia is not essential for the diagnosis of gastro-oesophageal reflux.

---

### FACTORS WHICH INCREASE THE CHANCE OF GASTRO-OESOPHAGEAL REFLUX

Raised intragastric pressure (large meals and volumes of liquids)

Lying and stooping

Obesity

Pregnancy

Gastric surgery

Alcohol and smoking

Scleroderma

Hiatus hernia with loss of intra-abdominal oesophagus

---

# 2

# Dysphagia

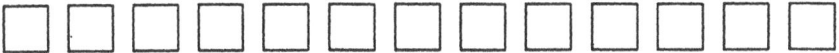

*The term dysphagia should be restricted to when solids or liquids will not pass from the mouth to stomach or do so only after an abnormal delay.* There may be accompanying retrosternal pain but this is not invariable.

## PHARYNGEAL DYSPHAGIA

Dysphagia occurring almost immediately the patient attempts to transfer food from the mouth to pharynx is likely to be due to one of the following:

– pharyngeal pouch
  pharyngo-oesophageal web
  postcricoid carcinoma
  neuromuscular disease

### Pharyngeal pouch

Characteristically there is discomfort in the throat at the start of swallowing with return to the mouth of some of the food or liquid. This can often be precipitated by change in position of the head and neck or pressure over the throat. Coughing due to aspiration into the larynx is common.

### *Management*

Diagnosis is by barium swallow. The radiologist should be asked to concentrate on the first phase of swallowing.

9

Explanation and reassurance that the condition is benign is often all that is required.

Surgery is indicated when aspiration is the major problem.

## Pharyngo-oesophageal web or stricture

Obstruction to swallowing solid food is the initial symptom but if the condition remains untreated, swallowing liquids will also eventually prove difficult. Aspiration occasionally occurs.

### Management

A barium swallow will usually establish the diagnosis.

All patients should be referred to a throat specialist for oesophagoscopy and dilatation of the stricture of resection of the web.

It is a misconception that all patients with this disorder have an iron deficiency anaemia. Nevertheless the haemoglobin and iron status should be measured and corrected when low.

Recurrence is common and long term follow-up is usually recommended because postcricoid carcinoma is a known complication.

## Postcricoid carcinoma

Rapid onset of dysphagia for solids and later for liquids *over a period of a few months* is characteristic of carcinoma in this region. Pain or discomfort not related to swallowing is common.

### Management

Early confirmation by barium swallow and endoscopy is essential.

A combination of surgery and radiotherapy or the latter alone is often curative.

## Neuromuscular disease

Paralysis of the soft palate and laryngopharyngeal muscles leads to aspiration of liquids and sometimes solids into the nasal and lower respiratory passages. This causes coughing and spluttering almost simultaneously with the initial phase of swallowing.

Major complications are pneumonia and lung abscess.

The condition is distinguished from mechanical obstruction by other symptoms and signs, particularly dysarthria. The commonest diseases involved are:

- motor neurone disease
  disseminated sclerosis
  recurrent stroke
  muscular dystrophies
  advanced Parkinsonism

## Management

The diagnosis of neuromuscular dysphagia is usually obvious but cineradiology of swallowing can sometimes provide additional helpful information.

There is most difficulty with liquids whereas puréed food is often taken with relatively little trouble.

When stroke or disseminated sclerosis is the cause, improvement may occur spontaneously. Seeking the help of a speech therapist to assist the patient to compensate for his or her bulbar disability may also be worthwhile.

If adequate nutrition cannot be maintained in a patient whose quality of life is otherwise satisfactory, a thin, highly flexible nasogastric tube can be used to give a balanced liquid diet. If there is sufficient support this treatment can be given at home.

## "Cortical dysphagia"

Another category of dysphagia is found in the old and mentally disturbed.

Patients can be observed to masticate food for several minutes but then seem to be incapable or unwilling to transfer the bolus beyond the upper pharynx. Eventually the food is spat out. Tablets are often treated similarly but fluids are taken without trouble, which helps distinguish the condition from many other forms of dysphagia.

## Management

The diagnosis is made on clinical evidence but, when doubt exists, a barium swallow will show that there is no mechanical lesion.

Nutrition may have to be maintained with a liquid diet. Encouragement should be given and the assistance of a speech therapist sought.

11

## Globus syndrome

A condition which must be distinguished from pharyngeal dysphagia is the globus syndrome.

This is best defined as a sensation in the throat which cannot be cleared. *There is little or no relationship to swallowing.* In some patients there are additional vague or bizarre somatic symptoms or clear evidence of anxiety and depression.

### *Management*

The larynx and pharynx must be examined as it is important to exclude organic pathology so that enthusiastic reassurance can be quickly given. The patient should be warned that the symptoms may persist for several months but that recovery eventually occurs spontaneously. Anxiety and depression when present should be treated appropriately.

## 'OESOPHAGEAL' DYSPHAGIA

As distinct from pharyngeal dysphagia, in oesophageal dysphagia there is a delay between starting to swallow and obstruction.

The common causes of 'oesophageal' dysphagia are:–

– benign peptic stricture
carcinoma of the oesophagus or gastric cardia
achalasia

## Benign peptic stricture

The vast majority of benign strictures are a complication of oesophagitis due to gastro-oesophageal reflux. Therefore a previous history of heartburn is common. Symptoms are initially intermittent often extending over a period of years. Even in advanced cases liquids tend to pass with little trouble. The appetite is preserved and weight is maintained. The patient often learns to induce regurgitation when solids block the strictured lumen.

### *Management*

*Barium swallow and endoscopy* are indicated in all patients complaining of *true* dysphagia.

Benign strictures appear on barium swallow in one of two forms. The more common are circumferential with smoothly tapering sides. They are usually less than 2 cm in length and tend to occur at the junction of the squamous and columnar epithelium. Less frequently the benign stricture appears as a short, smooth-walled cuff, but also involving the whole circumference of the distal oesophagus. This is the so-called Schatzski's ring and consists of fibrous tissue extending from the submucosal layers to the serosa. The epithelium has a normal appearance. Such lesions are considered to be the result of oesophagitis but why the epithelium itself is not overtly involved remains unclear.

Fibreoptic endoscopy is complementary to radiology and should be performed early. It makes possible a direct assessment of the nature and extent of the lesion. Furthermore, because it provides a means of obtaining biopsies and material for cytology, an accurate tissue diagnosis can be made in the majority of patients. This will assist in deciding about the course of future management, which is clearly dependent upon whether the stricture is benign or malignant. Whilst awaiting a definitive diagnosis the patient should be advised to eat *no* solids and maintain nutrition by taking fortified milk and soups. This will prevent complete obstruction and collection of debris in the oesophagus, thus facilitating endoscopic examination.

Benign peptic stricture having been confirmed, and distinguished from cancer by endoscopy, is best managed in the majority of cases by dilatation. The use of endoscopically positioned Eder Peustow or Celestin dilators has made this a safe and convenient treatment. The patient requires admission for only 24 hours. The number of dilations before achieving full patency of the oesophagus varies considerably. However, once established, recurrence of the stricture can usually be prevented by enthusiastic medical management of the underlying gastro-oesophageal reflux. In those patients where there is rapid and frequent recurrence, particularly if young, referral for resection of the stricture and antireflux surgery may be necessary.

## Carcinoma of oesophagus and gastric cardia

Cancers of the gastro-oesophageal junction are adeno-carcinomas whereas those of the middle and upper thirds of the oesophagus are usually squamous cell lesions. Both are commonest over the age of 60. Heavy smoking, excessive alcohol, oesophageal webs, achalasia, coeliac disease and teilosis are known predisposing factors.

In contrast to benign stricture a preceding history of heartburn or other symptoms of gastro-oesophageal reflux are rare. Dysphagia rapidly increases in severity and may be complete even for liquids in only a few weeks. Weight loss due to dysphagia and anorexia is almost invariable.

## Management

Barium swallow and fibreoptic oesophagoscopy are essential.

Unlike peptic strictures, which are virtually restricted to the distal oesophagus, carcinomas may occur at any site. Because they spread both longitudinally and circumferentially the narrowed segment is longer than in benign lesions, usually greater than 2 cm and the profile on barium swallow is often asymmetrical.

Endoscopic biopsy enables a tissue diagnosis to be made.

Treatment is by surgery or radiotherapy, but the relative merits of both are still undecided. Surgery is attempted for tumours involving the distal two thirds. In cases suitable for surgery the surgeon is usually able to obtain clearance of the lesion yet still be able to join the proximal oesophagus to stomach. In some patients this is not possible and a segment of colon has to be transplanted in order to provide continuity. It is claimed that radiotherapy gives results equal to those of surgery in cancers of the upper third of the oesophagus. Some centres have adopted a combined therapeutic approach but the results do not appear to be dramatically different from surgery alone.

A recent study has shown that lesions greater than 5 cm in length as measured on the barium swallow are almost invariably inoperable due to mediastinal spread. In such cases radiotherapy often proves of value as a palliative measure, temporarily relieving dysphagia and blood loss. An alternative palliative procedure for dysphagia is the insertion of a Mousseau Barbin or Celestin tube. These are wide bore tubes that can be passed orally down the oesophagus and through the stricture into the stomach. In the past, positioning of the tube has necessitated a gastrotomy but it can now be inserted without this operation by using special apparatus in conjunction with a fibreoptic endoscope. The tube permits a liquid diet which can maintain adequate nutrition for several months. Unfortunately, it is not without its own complications which include aspiration pneumonitis, blockage with food and tumour or erosion and perforation into the mediastinum

The overall prognosis is poor, with a five-year survival of approximately 10%.

## Achalasia

The absence or reduction of the Auerbach's plexus cells leads to an eventual absence of peristalsis and failure of the lower oesophageal sphincter to relax. The cause is obscure but viral and autoimmune aetiologies have been implicated.

14

Compared to benign and malignant strictures achalasia is a rare cause of dysphagia and tends to occur in younger age groups.

Attacks of severe spontaneous central chest pain, often occurring over several years, are frequently present before the patient presents with persistent dysphagia. Confusion with cardiac pain is common. Dysphagia eventually becomes the predominant symptom and occurs with both solids and liquids. By eating slowly, patients find that normal quantities can be taken because the oesophagus dilates and the weight of food within it eventually forces open the distal oesophageal sphincter. Rapid eating and lying down after a meal often lead to aspiration and violent coughing.

Swallowed air cannot enter the stomach in achalasia, which results in the absence of a gastric fundal air bubble on chest X-ray. This is sometimes a useful chance finding in patients who have been referred for chest X-ray because their predominant symptom is chest pain.

A condition termed *'diffuse oesophageal spasm'* is thought by some authorities to be a variant, or an evolutionary phase, of achalasia. Others believe it is a distinct entity. Spontaneous pain, often nocturnal, is a prominent symptom and the severity of dysphagia is variable.

## Management

As in all cases of true dysphagia patients suspected of having achalasia should be referred for barium swallow and fibreoptic endoscopy.

Radiology will show absent or reduced peristalsis of the oesophagus and non-relaxation of the lower oesophageal sphincter. By the time most patients are investigated the oesophagus will have dilated and developed an S-shaped configuration. Unlike the narrowed segment in carcinoma, which is long and irregular, in achalasia it is smooth and tapering. The condition of diffuse oesophageal spasm can be distinguished from classical achalasia by the presence of violent 'purposeless'' tertiary contractions which give the oesophagus a corkscrew appearance.

Endoscopy will confirm the diagnosis of achalasia and completely exclude peptic or carcinomatous stricture. An inflamed and oedematous mucosa is often seen, which is caused by irritation from stagnant food.

Until very recently drug therapy was unsatisfactory but studies now suggest that the calcium antagonist, nifedipine, 10–20 mg before meals may give benefit to some patients.

Surgery, however, is likely to be necessary eventually in the majority.

The operation of choice is cardiomyotomy (Heller's operation) which consists of cutting the muscle layers of the distal oesophagus down to the mucosa. Results are usually satisfactory but dysphagia may persist if the surgeon is too conservative. Because the operation disrupts the lower oesophageal sphincter, reflux of gastric contents commonly occurs and may itself become a clinical problem in some patients.

An alternative treatment to Heller's operation is dilatation of the lower oesophageal sphincter with inflatable bougies under radiological control. The procedure often has to be repeated and the overall results are not as satisfactory as those achieved by myotomy.

*Aspiration* into the lungs may be a major complication and is a definite indication for 'surgical' treatment. Whilst awaiting operation the patient should be instructed to take only small meals, not to eat just before retiring to bed and to raise the head end of the bed by approximately 6 inches (15 cm).

*Bleeding* from the congested and inflamed mucosa may cause anaemia, or more rarely, haematemesis and melaena.

An even more serious problem is the undoubted increased incidence of *carcinoma of the oesophagus*. Presentation is late and prognosis extremely poor. The clinician should be alerted to the possibility of malignancy by worsening dysphagia, anaemia, anorexia and weight loss. Unfortunately, there is little evidence that Heller's operation reduces the risk of developing cancer. As yet, there is no information about the value of long term endo-scopically monitored follow-up for 'early' detection of malignancy.

## Other disorders that cause dysphagia

The great majority of all patients with oesophageal dysphagia will be found to have peptic or carcinomatous stricture or achalasia.

Nevertheless, a number of other conditions may lead to dysphagia, although it is rarely the presenting or predominant symptom in these dis-orders. Such conditions include *scleroderma* and *dermatomyositis*, both of which are usually obvious from other characteristic features of the diseases. *Carcinoma of the bronchus* or *lymphoma* involving mediastinal nodes may sometimes cause dysphagia either by invasion or extrinsic pressure. Other signs are usually present and chest X-ray will clarify the situation. Pain whilst swallowing may also be caused by *candidiasis* of the oesophagus. The characteristic white lesions are also frequently present in the mouth and pharynx. It is most commonly found in diabetics and those taking steroids, antibiotics or cytotoxic drugs. It should be treated with nystatin or amphotericin B. Many drugs are capable of inducing oesophagitis and strictures, especially in the elderly. *All tablets* should be taken with a minimum of 100 ml of water to ensure they enter the stomach.

*It is important to distinguish true dysphagia (obstruction or delay in swallowing) from the sensation of 'a lump' which only comes on after a meal. The latter is usually due to uncomplicated oesophagitis. True dysphagia demands urgent investigation whereas uncomplicated oesophagitis does not (see Chapter 1).*

---

*Distinction between benign and malignant oesophageal strictures*

| Benign | Malignant |
|---|---|
| Previous heartburn common | Previous pain uncommon |
| Often intermittent dysphagia for many months | Progressive dysphagia for a few weeks |
| Weight and appetite maintained | Weight loss and anorexia |

---

*The sensation of a lump stuck in the chest or throat*

- Soon after eating a meal – gastro-oesophageal reflux
- Whilst swallowing – stricture (peptic or carcinoma)
- Not related to eating – globus syndrome or laryngeal disease

17

# 3

# Nausea and Vomiting

Nausea and vomiting can be subdivided into acute, persistent and episodic. Nausea and vomiting are usually closely associated. The former often occurs alone, though it usually precedes vomiting. Vomiting without nausea is rare.

## ACUTE VOMITING

Acute vomiting precedes many disorders. It is usually accompanied by symptoms or signs facilitating diagnosis. Thus, the diarrhoea and malaise which accompany vomiting in *acute viral* or *bacterial gastroenteritis* make the diagnosis obvious. Nausea and profound anorexia rather than vomiting is typical of *viral hepatitis*, usually preceding jaundice by several days. Acute vomiting sometimes accompanies *biliary colic, pancreatitis, renal colic* and even *myocardial infarction*. The mechanism is not clear but it is thought to be due to non-specific response to pain. In the latter two conditions it can cause a confusing diversion from the diagnosis.

*Acute vestibulitis* and *cerebrovascular lesions* cause severe vertigo, nausea and frequently vomiting. Raised intracranial pressure due to *malignant hypertension, intracranial tumour* and *intracranial haemorrhage* are well recognised causes of vomiting. Nausea is often absent in this latter triad.

## PERSISTENT VOMITING

Conditions characterised by persistent vomiting usually have accompanying symptoms simplifying diagnosis. Successful management consists of treating the cause.

### Gastrointestinal diseases

*Pyloric stenosis*, due to *chronic duodenal ulcer* or *carcinoma of the stomach* gives rise to persistent large-volume vomiting. Undigested food eaten hours before is identifiable, and a succussion splash may be produced by vigorous palpation of the upper abdomen. *Intestinal obstruction* is another cause. It is characteristically accompanied by colic and abdominal distension. Pyloric stenosis and intestinal obstruction require urgent hospital admission for correction of electrolyte imbalance, gastric aspiration and usually surgical intervention.

### Non-gastrointestinal diseases

Nausea and vomiting is a common feature in the first trimester of *pregnancy*. It is most severe first thing in the morning and occasionally at night. The condition rarely gives rise to dehydration and usually resolves by the end of the first trimester. Eating dry toast or biscuits before rising is usually of help, drug therapy very rarely being necessary. Patients may forget to mention the possibility of pregnancy. Examination of the breasts and the history of amenorrhoea will avoid unnecessary investigation.

*Drug therapy*, especially if recently prescribed, should be suspected as a potential cause of nausea and vomiting. The most commonly implicated are cytotoxics, anti-inflammatory drugs and some antibiotics, morphine, codeine and their derivatives have the same effect. Digoxin is worth remembering especially in the elderly and in patients with renal impairment.

Vomiting may be prominent in *metabolic* and *endocrine* disorders. Vomiting in association with muscle weakness, depression and constipation should raise the suspicion of *hypercalcaemia. Addison's disease*, commonly, and *thyrotoxicosis*, less frequently, present with unexplained vomiting. The underlying cause in Addison's disease is thought to be hyponatraemia, because patients with *sodium deficiency* from other disorders also suffer from nausea and vomiting. *Hepatic* and *renal failure are frequently complicated by persistent vomiting*.

## EPISODIC VOMITING

There are many conditions of diverse aetiology which give rise to episodic vomiting. The attacks are frequently brief and resolve spontaneously so the patient often does not seek advice until several episodes have occurred.

## Psychogenic vomiting

When periodic nausea and vomiting occur in apparent isolation, by far the commonest cause is *psychogenic* disturbance. Certain susceptible individuals react to acute stress by vomiting. When there is a prolonged stressful unresolved situation vomiting can become a chronic or recurrent problem.

If it is suspected that stress is a cause of periodic vomiting and it is not readily volunteered by the patient, it is a good idea to interview relatives and friends. Features of organic disease are absent and very rarely is there any significant electrolyte disturbance or weight loss. Accompanying anxiety and depression may be relieved by vomiting. This may be because of the increased sympathy and attention that this physical symptom arouses. It is not uncommon for patients who have suffered from previous organic gastrointestinal disease to have alimentary psychogenic symptoms. It is very important to exclude recurrence of the original problem in such patients. In children cyclical vomiting can occur as a result of domestic tension or problems at school.

A small proportion of women suffer from vomiting at a certain stage of their menstrual cycle. It has not been clearly established whether the cause is hormonal or psychological.

The crucial factor of management in psychogenic vomiting is identification and treatment of the underlying cause. Antidepressants or tranquilizers may be of some help.

## Anorexia nervosa

A quite separate group of individuals who present with episodic vomiting are those who suffer from anorexia nervosa. The vast majority are female in the age group 14 – 30 years. Diagnosis relies on eliciting typical features from patient, friends and relatives. These include the patient's distorted view of her body, size and image, weight loss, amenorrhoea, strict avoidance of carbohydrates and overactivity. In addition to vomiting the patient may practise diuretic and laxative abuse (Chapter 11). Management is very difficult and hinges on getting the patient to accept a more normal view of her body image, and a balanced view of food. A commonly adopted policy is to get the patient to gradually increase her intake and weight for simple rewards. The setting of weight targets for specific deadlines is also important as a measure of success.

Depression and psychosis may need to be treated as well.

A related problem is *bulimia nervosa*, when the patient gorges herself and then induces copious vomiting as a result of guilt and gross abdominal distension. Weight loss is not usually such a significant feature. Referral for psychiatric treatment is required in most cases.

## Alcohol

Nausea and especially vomiting and retching on first rising are common symptoms of alcohol abuse. Patients almost invariably fail to realize or refuse to admit that alcohol may be the cause of the problem. Patients may often be unnecessarily investigated unless alcohol is borne in mind. A positive history is rarely forthcoming and friends and relatives should always be interviewed before investigations. The presence of coexistent diarrhoea, which is also common with alcohol abuse, may increase the pressure to investigate. Admission to hospital, and thus enforced abstinence causing cessation of symptoms, is proof positive as to the cause. The finding of an elevated serum $\gamma$ -glutamyl transferase supports this diagnosis. The mechanism causing the vomiting seems to be as much due to central nervous system disturbance as gastric irritation.

## Migraine

Nausea and vomiting may be a prominent feature of migraine. The characteristic headache allied to the prodromal symptoms such as teichopsia and hemianopia usually make the diagnosis certain. A minority of patients suffer from abdominal pain with migraine and this may stimulate gastrointestinal investigation.

## Menière's and cerebellar disease

The vertigo of Menière's disease is often accompanied by vomiting. Vertigo with vomiting may also occur in disseminated sclerosis, but usually there are additional neurological symptoms.

## Peptic disease

*Recurrent vomiting in the absence of pain is very rare in peptic ulcer. Gastro-oesophageal reflux*, leading to regurgitation of stomach contents into the mouth, may lead to vomiting without nausea. Careful history taking will elicit the true sequence of events. Vomiting of gastric contents, often containing large amounts of bile, occurs in a small but significant number of patients who have undergone *partial gastrectomy*. It tends to decrease with time and rarely warrants further surgery.

## EPISODIC VOMITING

- Psychogenic causes are commonest
- Vomiting with amenorrhoea and weight loss in adolescence – consider anorexia nervosa
- Vomiting soon after waking in the morning usually due to alcohol abuse
- Vomiting without abdominal pain is rarely due to peptic ulcer

# 4

# Uncomplicated Peptic Ulcer

The commonest sites of peptic ulceration are the duodenum and stomach. It occurs less frequently in the oesophagus as a complication of gastro-oesophageal reflux and at the anastomosis of stomach and intestinal mucosa following gastric surgery. It is a worldwide disease. In the United Kingdom duodenal ulcer has an incidence in men of more than two per 1000 and in women of 0.62 per 1000. Gastric ulcer is less common, the figures being 0.53 per 1000 for men and 0.31 per 1000 in women. It has been estimated that at some time in their life one in five men and one in ten women develop a peptic ulcer. Although both duodenal and gastric ulcer are very common diseases it seems likely that their incidence has decreased during the past 25 years. Gastric ulcers are more common in social classes 4 and 5 (UK classification) than in those with professional and managerial occupations. Duodenal ulcer is distributed equally throughout the population.

## PATHOGENESIS

Ulceration occurs when the mucosa breaks down under the erosive effect of acid and pepsin. The mechanisms that predispose or lead to this imbalance between mucosal resistance and erosive forces are not fully understood.

Traditionally gastric acid and pepsin, the 'attacking' factors, are considered to be of major importance in duodenal ulcer. This is because many patients with duodenal ulcer have excessive or prolonged secretion of gastric acid and pepsin under basal conditions and following stimulation by pentagastrin, food or antral distension.

Rapid emptying of the stomach and failure to coordinate this with adequate quantities of alkaline pancreatic secretions also occurs in some patients.

In the vast majority of patients with duodenal ulcer an excess of gastrin *per se* is *not* the cause of abnormal gastric secretion. Nevertheless there could be a subtle imbalance between the stimulation of gastrin and the inhibitory hormones secretion and somatostatin.

Despite these abnormalities of gastric secretion it seems improbable that they are the total cause of duodenal ulcer and study is now being directed towards possible defects in the duodenal mucosa.

By contrast with duodenal ulcer, gastric ulcer is not associated with abnormally high levels of gastric acid and, indeed, hypochlorhydria is common. There has therefore been a longstanding suggestion that faulty mucosal resistance is the major pathogenic component in this condition.

Thus, in both gastric and duodenal ulcer there might be either a quantitative or qualitative defect in the 'protective' layer of mucus. Alternatively, there could be a primary defect in epithelial cell regeneration or a predisposition to attack from acid and pepsin. Deficiency of epidermal growth factor or prostaglandins could be possible mechanisms for these pathogenic processes.

Recurrent duodenogastric reflux and gastric stasis are associated with stomach ulcer. Both phenomena would allow noxious substances to have prolonged contact with the mucosa.

Why only small areas of the gastroduodenal mucosa ulcerate is not clear. It has been suggested that relative ischaemia may be important and that the lesser curve of the stomach and first part of the duodenum could be particularly vulnerable, owing to a deficient collateral circulation.

## AETIOLOGICAL FACTORS

### Genetic

Duodenal and gastric ulcers occur more commonly in those with blood group O and certain HLA tissue antigens. There is an increased family incidence in both diseases.

### Diet

An unrefined masticatory diet may protect from duodenal ulcer.

### Smoking

Smokers suffer from peptic ulcer more commonly than non-smokers.

## Drugs

Aspirin and other non-steroidal anti-inflammatory drugs have been implicated as a cause of gastric ulcer, but unequivocal evidence is lacking.

## Psychological factors

Although emotional stress profoundly influences alimentary tract function there is very little evidence that it is an important cause of chronic ulceration in man.

## Virus infection

There is a possible relationship between duodenal ulcer and herpes simplex infection.

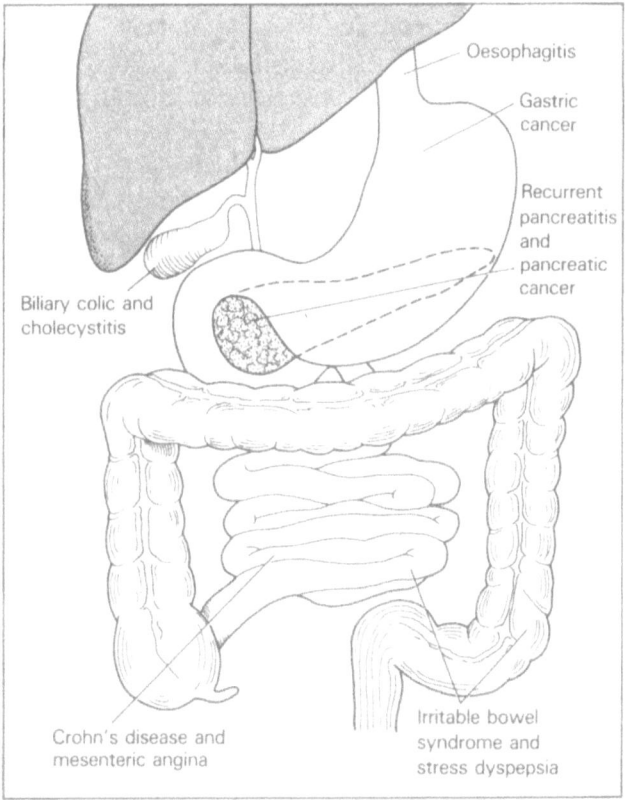

**Figure 4.1**  Diseases that may be confused with peptic ulcer (from Lancaster-Smith, M. (1983) *Peptic Ulcer*. (London: Update Publications))

## CLINICAL FEATURES

*Pain* is by far the most common symptom. It is most commonly experienced in the epigastrium and the site is often identified by the patient pointing with a single finger. Radiation is to the chest, back and hypochondria. Pain is described as gnawing, knife-like or severe hunger. Intensity does *not* correlate with size or incipient complications. Food may precipitate or relieve symptoms. Antacids more consistently relieve symptoms but this is incomplete in more than 50%. Pain that wakes a patient in the early hours of the morning is highly suggestive of duodenal ulcer.

*Vomiting* may occur and often gives rapid relief from pain. It does not necessarily indicate pyloric stenosis.

*Heartburn* is a common associated symptom in patients with duodenal ulcer.

Peptic ulcer symptoms occur in bouts lasting from several days to several weeks, interspersed with remissions of many months.

Slight weight loss may occur, but profound reduction in weight and anorexia are *not* features of peptic disease and are highly likely to be due to gastric cancer.

It is impossible to distinguish clinically between gastric and duodenal ulcer. In uncomplicated cases the only physical sign is tenderness in the epigastrium, but during remission even this may be absent.

## MANAGEMENT

The aims of management are:

relief of symptoms
healing of the ulcer
prevention of relapse
prevention of complications

### Initial approach

It is impractical to investigate every patient with symptoms compatible with peptic ulcer. When peptic ulcer seems likely in the under 40 age group it is reasonable to give an initial course of antacids or an ulcer-healing drug (see below) combined with general advice.

### Advice to patient

The salient points are as follows:

Try to eliminate or reduce daily 'stress'.

A few days away from work at the start of treatment may be very helpful.

Three normal meals per day are advisable. 'Gastric' diets do not enhance healing.

Alcohol in moderation (two drinks per day) will not delay healing but often seems to precipitate symptoms.

Coffee should be avoided.

Smoking delays healing and should be stopped. If this is impossible, smoking before going to bed must be strongly discouraged as it will negate nocturnal $H_2$-blockade.

Many patients will achieve good results with this approach and, providing attacks are infrequent, subsequent attacks may be dealt with in a similar fashion. All patients must be warned that peptic ulcer is a recurrent problem for which, as yet, there is no definite cure.

If symptoms recur rapidly and frequently or are not adequately relieved, investigation to confirm the diagnosis and exclude alternative pathologies is appropriate.

### Confirmation of diagnosis

*Barium meal* is still the most commonly requested investigation in those suspected of peptic ulcer. However, about 25% of ulcers will escape detection in most centres. *Endoscopy* is less likely to miss peptic ulcer and over 90% will be identified in most established units. *But if a barium meal shows duodenal ulcer endoscopy is not necessary.*

By contrast, when recurrent symptoms are compatible with peptic disease but radiology fails to confirm ulceration, endoscopy should be considered. It may well reveal a posterior wall gastric ulcer or duodenitis. The latter condition is closely associated with duodenal ulcer and almost certainly the same causal factors and management principles are applicable.

Similarly, when a gastric ulcer is found by barium meal endoscopy with biopsy is indicated to exclude stomach cancer. In some areas this will not be immediately available, in which case gastroscopy should be reserved for patients in whom symptoms or repeat X-rays indicate failure to heal after a 6-week course of treatment.

### $H_2$-Antagonists

The search for a means of suppressing gastric acid secretion in peptic ulcer was stimulated by the fact that many patients with duodenal ulcer are hypersecretors and operations that reduce acid output are very successful in healing ulcers. Histamine has long been considered the most important final mediator of parietal cell stimulation. However, conventional antihistamines ($H_1$-antagonists) have no significant action on gastric secretion and it was therefore postulated that there are different histamine receptors on the parietal cells. We now know these as $H_2$-receptors.

## Cimetidine

Cimetidine (Tagamet) inhibits gastric secretion, both basal secretion and that in response to all stimuli. It is rapidly absorbed and in the fasting state peak blood levels are found at 1 – 2 hours. Renal excretion of the unchanged drug is rapid. The blood half-life of cimetidine is of the order of 2 hours. However, by taking the tablet with meals, which delays absorption, therapeutic blood levels are prolonged.

There is overwhelming evidence from a large number of trials throughout the world that cimetidine rapidly relieves symptoms in the great majority of patients with duodenal ulcer and that healing is enhanced. Approximately 80% of duodenal ulcers heal during a 4 – 6-week course of treatment compared to about 35% that heal on placebo. The most commonly used regime has been 200 mg t.d.s. and 400 mg nocte, but recent studies suggest that this can be simplified to 400 mg b.d. without loss of efficacy.

Cimetidine also relieves symptoms in gastric ulcer and healing, while less impressive than in duodenal ulcer, can be expected in about 70% of those taking the drug compared with about 40% placebo healing.

Why a considerable proportion of duodenal and gastric ulcers fail to heal with cimetidine is not clear, but there is evidence that these patients have higher basal and peak acid outputs than do those whose ulcers heal.

Considering that more than 15 million people throughout the world have received this drug, reports of unwanted effects have been very rare. They include drowsiness and confusion, particularly in the elderly and those with renal and hepatic impairment, gynaecomastia, impotence, diarrhoea and skin rashes. Cimetidine inhibits hepatic cytochrome C450 which results in higher than normal blood levels of drugs such as phenytoin, propranolol and warfarin when they are taken concurrently. Because reduction of gastric acidity encourages bacterial growth, with the formation of potentially carcinogenic nitrites in the gastric lumen, there has been concern that the use of $H_2$-antagonists may predispose to stomach cancer. As yet there is no evidence from extensive animal work that this is so.

## Ranitidine

Ranitidine (Zantac) is the only other $H_2$-antagonist currently available. It has the same pharmacological action on gastric secretion as cimetidine but, weight for weight, is approximately four times more potent. Given in a dose of 150 mg twice daily it suppresses gastric acid secretion to a greater extent than cimetidine 200 mg t.d.s. and 400 mg nocte. Although this may improve compliance it probably has little additional clinical benefit.

Trials on patients with both duodenal and gastric ulcer have shown healing rates for ranitidine strikingly similar to those previously found with cimetidine.

Ranitidine's main advantage over cimetidine is its apparent lack of side-effects and absence of drug interactions. The chief disadvantage is that at the moment it costs more than cimetidine.

## Antacids

For many years antacids have been the mainstay of ulcer treatment. Until recently no healing effect had been shown and their efficacy was based upon symptom relief. When an antacid is used in this way most patients tend to take it only when symptoms occur and vary the dose and frequency accordingly. However, it may be more logical to advise taking the preparation regularly $1\frac{1}{2}$ – 2 hours after completing a meal, before going to bed and at other times when necessary, as this would reduce the high peaks of intraluminal gastric acidity. Numerous studies have demonstrated that a liquid antacid is significantly better than antacid tablets for pain relief. It should be remembered that the multitude of antacid preparations available have widely varying buffering capacity (Table 4.1).

The neutralizing effect of 30 ml of Maalox, a combination of magnesium and aluminium compounds, taken 1 and 3 hours after a meal is about the same as that of cimetidine 400 mg taken with the meal.

## Side-effects

The major advantage of antacid therapy is the relative lack of unwanted effects. Sodium bicarbonate, although providing very rapid relief, should not be used on a long term basis because it is readily absorbed and can cause significant alkalosis. Aluminium salts often constipate and magnesium salts lead to diarrhoea. Combinations are therefore advisable. Calcium-containing salts rapidly neutralize hydrochloric acid but should be avoided as calcium stimulates gastrin release and leads to rebound hypersecretion of acid.

31

| Antacid | Neutralizing capacity (ml of 0.1N HCl) per 10 ml of antacid or per tablet |
|---|---|
| *Liquids* | |
| Magnesium trisilicate BPC | 220 |
| Aluminium hydroxide gel BPC | 255 |
| Antasil | 428 |
| Maalox | 233 |
| Polycrol forte gel | 230 |
| Mylanta | 220 |
| Asilone gel | 194 |
| Asilone suspension | 301 |
| Mucaine | 294 |
| Liquid Gaviscon | 55 |
| *Tablets* | |
| Magnesium trisilicate BPC | 45 |
| Aludrox | 142 |
| Antasil | 204 |
| Maalox | 240 |
| Polycrol forte | 100 |
| Asilone | 105 |
| Gaviscon | 15 |
| Nulacin | 93 |
| Gelusil | 65 |
| Actal | 84 |

**Table 4.1**   The buffering capacities of proprietary antacids

## Bismuth

Tripotassium dicitratobismuthate in a colloidal alkalinated solution (De-nol) promotes healing of peptic ulcers. Five recent trials using endoscopic assessment found from 74 to 94% of ulcers healed after 4 – 6 weeks of 'active' treatment, compared with the 13 – 21% that healed on placebo. Similarly, in three trials on gastric ulcers the bismuth preparation healed 85 – 90% after 4 weeks' treatment compared to 30 – 35% on placebo. In other trials healing rates with De-nol were comparable to those achieved with cimetidine (Tagamet). The volume most commonly used was 20 ml per day in divided doses.

The mode of action of De-nol is not clear but is thought to include the formation of a protective film over the ulcer due to precipitation of bismuth with the proteinaceous exudate, stimulation of mucus and an antipepsin activity. It has no significant side-effects but many patients find the ammoniacal smell difficult to tolerate. *This problem may now have been overcome by the production of a tablet formulation which seems to be equally efficacious*.

## Sucralfate

Sucralfate has an antipepsin action and allegedly also forms a protective layer over damaged gastroduodenal mucosa. Trials in Japan and the USA have shown healing rates in duodenal and gastric ulcer comparable to those achieved with cimetidine, but a small radiologically monitored study in Wales showed no significant benefit in patients with gastric ulcer.

## Carbenoxolone

This drug is derived from glycyrrhizinic acid which occurs naturally in liquorice. It has no significant antisecretory action and is effective because it 'strengthens' the gastroduodenal mucosa. It does so by increasing mucus production and prolonging mucosal cell life. For duodenal ulcer the preparation used is Duogastrone, in which the carbenoxolone is encapsulated and hence delivered in high concentration to the duodenal mucosa. Five recent trials monitored by endoscopy have shown that a 4 – 6-week course heals 60 – 75% of duodenal ulcers, comapred to 19 – 48% placebo healing. Similar healing rates for gastric ulcer, using Biogastrone, were found by Doll as early as 1962 and have been confirmed in numerous subsequent trials.

### Side-effects

Fluid and sodium retention, hypokalaemia and hypertension due to a mineralocorticoid activity are major unwanted effects. These are reduced by restricting the daily dose to 150 mg but thiazide diuretics and potassium supplements are now prescribed prophylactically by some practitioners. If these are not given, the patient's cardiovascular status and electrolytes should be reviewed weekly. The risk is greatest in the elderly and with the advent of alternative drugs the use of carbenoxolone in this age group is no longer advised.

## Deglycyrrhizinized liquorice

Trials with both Caved-S and Ulcedal have given equivocal results. It seems likely that both are less effective in healing ulcers than carbenoxolone.

## Pirenzepine

This is a new tricyclic drug which is said to have an anticholinergic action mainly on the stomach and has given promising results under trial conditions. Whether it will be sufficiently free of side-effects to compete with $H_2$-antagonists remains to be seen.

## Trimipramine

The antidepressant drug trimipramine (Surmontil) has been found to have a significant healing effect on both gastric and duodenal ulcer. The mode of action is unclear but it seems that there may be either an anticholinergic action or direct reduction of parietal cell sensitivity. The use of trimipramine is likely to be limited by side-effects, such as drowsiness and blurred vision.

## Anticholinergic drugs

Drugs in this group, which include atropine (Eumydrin), glycopyrronium (Robinul), hyoscine (Buscopan), poldine (Nacton) and propantheline (Pro-Banthine), when given intravenously or in large oral doses significantly reduce gastric secretion by competitively inhibiting acetycholine at postganglionic nerve endings. However, when the drugs are used in this way side-effects such as blurred vision, dry mouth and drowsiness are inevitable.

## Prostaglandins

Prostaglandins are a group of naturally occurring cyclic fatty acids which have a very wide range of activity. One group inhibits gastric secretion and has an intrinsic cytoprotective action. A synthetic analogue, methylprostaglandin $E_2$, has healed gastric and duodenal ulcers in preliminary studies but further trials are needed before its place can be assessed.

## PREVENTION OF RECURRENCE

That peptic ulcer is a relapsing disease has been emphasized in recent years by the very high recurrence rates found in endoscopically monitored long term maintenance trials. These studies have also clearly shown that recurrence of ulceration, seen endoscopically, is considerably more common than symptomatic relapse.

Endoscopy has confirmed, perhaps not surprisingly, that complete healing of a gastric ulcer leads to a longer remission than when healing is incomplete.

The length of the initial course of cimetidine used has no influence on the recurrence rate after the drug is stopped, the incidence being the same following either a 6-week or 12- month full-dose course of treatment.

## Prophylaxis

Approximately 80% of patients maintained on placebo after their duodenal ulcer has been healed by cimetidine have a recurrence of ulceration within 6 – 12 months. This compares with a 20% relapse rate over the same period in those taking a maintenance dose of cimetidine. It seems that 400 mg cimetidine nocte is adequate and that even better results can be achieved with ranitidine 150 mg nocte. The recurrence of gastric ulcer is also reduced by long term maintenance with both cimetidine and ranitidine, but the optimum dosage and regime are not yet clear.

None of the other ulcer-healing preparations has an established role in prevention of recurrence.

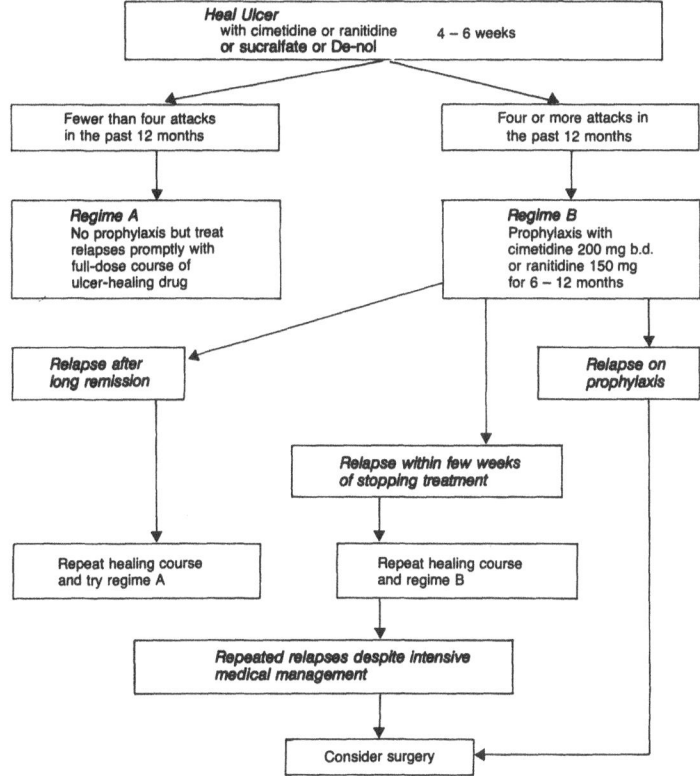

**Figure 4.2**  Selection of patients with peptic ulcer for prophylaxis

## A long term problem

Despite recent innovations peptic ulcer remains a long term problem for the majority of patients. It is not possible to be dogmatic about the choice of a long term regimen (see Table 4.1). Almost certainly many patients keep themselves free of symptoms by the occasional very short-term use of antacids or, indeed, other more 'potent' agents. Others, with long asymptomatic remissions, will happily take a full 6-week course of an ulcer-healing drug whenever symptoms return. A third group, usually because of the 'severity' of their disease, may reasonably be selected for low-dose maintenance therapy after the initial healing course. Severity in this context is difficult to define but the criteria include:

(1)   a bleed on more than one occasion,

(2)   a penetrating ulcer,

(3)   an average of more than four relapses per year (the cost of four 6-week healing courses of cimetidine is roughly equivalent to that of a single healing course and 46 weeks' low-dose maintenance)

In addition, the old and those suffering from other diseases, who might be embarrassed by a complication of their ulcer, should also seriously be considered for long term maintenance.

The length of long term treatment is impossible to define. The course of the disease varies widely from one patient to another and all that can be advised is occasional trial withdrawal of maintenance treatment to see if it is still required.

Failure to achieve a response with full-dose courses of ulcer healing preparations or frequent relapse whilst on low-dose maintenance are indications to consider surgery.

## LONG TERM PROGNOSIS

The eventual outcome and likely need for surgery in a patient with duodenal ulcer is extremely difficult to predict at initial presentation. Furthermore, studies on large groups of patients have revealed a widely varying prognosis and operation rate.

Fry, studying patients who in the main did not require hospital referral and therefore presumably had relatively mild disease, found that 90% were asymptomatic or little troubled by their disease 10 years after diagnosis. Symptoms in this group reached a peak during the seventh year after onset. In contrast patients referred to hospital who are, therefore, likely to have more severe disease, appear to have a less favourable prognosis.

Scandinavian studies in such groups have shown that within 13 years more than 20% had received an operation and that in those followed for 18 – 33 years, 43% had undergone surgery. At the same stages of follow-up only 37% and 20% respectively were asymptomatic.

Gastric ulcer appears to have a comparable long term prognosis. In a large group of Scandinavian patients reviewed 18 – 33 years after diagnosis, 32% had required surgery, 15% had continued to experience severe symptoms and only 29% were asymptomatic.

## POINTS TO REMEMBER

### New case with possible ulcer symptoms

- Advice on diet and smoking

- Warn patient that he is likely to have recurrences for several years

- Take antacids in sufficient quantities to relieve symptoms

- Follow-up after 2 weeks to assess progress

### Persistent/recurrent symptoms

- Refer for barium meal studies

- If gastric ulcer is shown then refer for endoscopy (if available) to exclude gastric cancer

- If duodenal ulcer no need for endoscopy

- A spell away from work to facilitate initial treatment

- Avoidance of stress

- $H_2$-antagonists or sucralfate or De-No1

- In gastric ulcer repeat barium meal or endoscopy after 6 weeks' treatment to check healing

### Continuing care

- Avoid factors likely to exacerbate disease such as smoking, dietary indiscretion and excess alcohol

- Use ulcer-healing treatment promptly as soon as symptoms return

- If frequent recurrence, consider long term low-dose $H_2$-antagonists

## Referral to specialist

– After barium meal if diagnosis in doubt or treatment unsuccessful

– For reassurance of patient and relatives, especially when symptoms keep recurring

– For possible surgery when persistent enthusiastic medical care has failed

## Long term care

– Peptic ulcer patients require long term care and arrangements must be made for this

– Patients should know how to treat themselves but also when to report to their physician, e.g. if pain changes or becomes persistent and unrelieved, if vomiting becomes prominent or if haematemesis or melaena occur

– A practice register of peptic ulcer patients is helpful in plotting the natural history and checking follow-up

– All ulcer patients after surgery must have annual full blood count to check for possible occurrence of anaemia

# 5

# Complicated Peptic Ulcer

## BLEEDING

In Britain bleeding from the upper gastrointestinal tract accounts for approximately 25 000 admissions to hospital and 2500 deaths each year. Peptic ulcers cause about 55% of acute upper gastrointestinal bleeds. Haemorrhage is the commonest event to complicate peptic ulcer and is the most frequent cause of death attributable to the disease. It results in more than twice as many deaths as perforation.

Long term follow-up studies have shown that approximately 20% of patients with duodenal ulcer bleed over a 20 year period. However, the risk of haemorrhage is greatest in the first year of the disease. Haemorrhage also tends to be a more common presenting feature in elderly patients than in younger age groups. Patients who experience haemorrhage have a twofold chance of future bleeding compared with patients who have not bled.

Those with blood group O bleed more frequently and at a younger age than patients with other blood groups. In contrast, inability to secrete ABO(H) blood group substances by exocrine glands is not associated with an increased propensity to haemorrhage. There is no doubt that aspirin causes micro-bleeding from the gastric mucosa. In contrast there is little sound evidence that aspirin taken in moderation precipitates bleeding from peptic ulcers. Heavy intake, i.e. more than four doses per week for at least 3 months, does cause a significant increase in the incidence of haemorrhage from the upper gastrointestinal tract.

## Assessment of severity

Most patients who have a haematemesis are in no doubt that the blood was vomited. However, blood discovered in the mouth may have originated from the postnasal space or lower respiratory tract. This can cause confusion unless time is taken to elicit an accurate history. The haematemesis may consist either of fresh blood mixed with gastric fluid or changed blood in the form of 'coffee ground'. *All such patients should be referred to hospital for admission because haematemesis indicates a recent haemorrhage*.

The patient's estimate of how much blood has been vomited is seldom helpful in assessing the true severity of the bleed. In contrast, vomitus saved by the patient or produced in the presence of the practitioner is a useful guide. Haematemesis may be accompanied by melaena but because most patients who vomit blood rapidly seek medical attention, it is not always initially present. If no stool has been passed rectal examination may reveal melaena. This can sometimes be helpful when there is doubt about the validity of haematemesis. Melaena without haematemesis often indicates a less severe bleed. However, *when melaena is fresh or has been present for 3 days or less, admission to hospital is still required*. A patient who passed melaena more than 3 days previously, providing he is not anaemic and remains otherwise healthy, does not necessarily require urgent admission but early investigation is nevertheless advisable. Confusion can sometimes arise in patients taking iron- or bismuth-containing preparations because they both cause darkening of the stool. Neither gives a positive occult blood test.

Physical signs following gastrointestinal haemorrhage are often misleading and frequently underestimate the true blood loss. Pallor of the skin, a pulse rate of greater than 100 per minute and a systolic blood pressure of less than 100 mmHg or a diastolic pressure of less than 65 mgHg indicate the need for blood transfusion. These measurements taken with the patient lying down may not always detect hypovolaemia. Thus, if normal they should be repeated with the patient sitting or standing. A drop in pressure and rise in pulse rate are indications of a significant reduction in blood volume. On admission to hospital estimation of the central venous pressure will provide an even more accurate means of assessing the degree of hypovolaemia. A haemoglobin concentration of less than 9 g/100 ml suggests severe haemorrhage. However, normal levels do not exclude this because vasoconstriction can maintain a misleadingly high haemoglobin concentration.

## The site of bleeding

*In acute gastrointestinal bleeding, establishing the cause of bleeding is secondary to assessment of severity and resuscitation.*

## Clinical features

Although a previous peptic ulcer history may be helpful it does not prove that there is an existing ulcer or that it is the site of haemorrhage. Furthermore, a significant proportion of patients who bleed from peptic ulcers have no history of dyspepsia. Aspirin and anti-inflammatory drugs cause gastrointestinal haemorrhage, but the role of aspirin in clinically apparent gastrointestinal haemorrhage has almost certainly been over-stated. A history of aspirin consumption during the previous 48 hours is therefore probably irrelevant and does not help in diagnosing the nature of the lesion. The evidence that steroids cause significant gastrointestinal haemorrhage is even more tenuous. Alcohol abuse may be a factor in patients with peptic ulcer, gastric erosions, varices or oesophageal tears. In the latter, which is not always alcohol induced, haematemesis is usually preceded by an initial vomit that produces no blood.

Although cutaneous signs of chronic liver disease, ascites and splenomegaly suggest the possibility of variceal bleeding, it should be remembered that peptic ulcer and gastric erosions are also commonly associated with cirrhosis. A history or signs of recent weight loss, anorexia or a mass in the epigastrium points to a diagnosis of stomach cancer. Carcinoma of the caecum may give rise to melaena. A palpable mass in the right iliac fossa and a change in bowel habit are other features of this disease.

The great majority of patients with gastrointestinal haemorrhage have a local lesion in the gut. Nevertheless, in a small proportion more generalized disease is responsible. These include bleeding diatheses, leukaemia, polyarteritis nodosa, Henoch–Schönlein purpura and chronic renal failure. Other features of these disorders are usually present or obvious after simple routine investigations.

## PERFORATION

Perforation of a peptic ulcer is considerably less common than haemorrhage, occurring in less than 5% of patients. The perforation rate is greater for gastric ulcers but because the incidence of duodenal ulcer is higher most perforations are a complication of the latter. The vast majority of duodenal ulcers that perforate are positioned on the anterior surface of the first part. Perforation of duodenal ulcer appears to be particularly common in men;

the reasons for this are not clear. Admissions for perforated peptic ulcer are declining. The main reason for this, in respect of duodenal ulcer, is the overall decrease in incidence. The same applies to gastric ulcer but, in addition, during the past two decades there has been a reduction in the proportion of gastric ulcers which perforate. The declining incidence of perforation has been accompanied by an increase in the average age of those affected.

It is impossible to predict on clinical evidence which ulcers are likely to perforate and indeed up to 20% have suffered from no significant dyspepsia prior to the perforation.

## Clinical features

*The predominant symptom is sudden severe epigastric pain*. The patient usually lies very still, in the supine position, taking shallow breaths because all movement exacerbates the pain. This may remain localized to the epigastrium but often continuing leakage of gastric and duodenal contents gives rise to more generalized peritoneal irritation. On palpation of the abdomen there is 'board-like rigidity'. Bowel sounds are absent and liver dullness may be diminished. Systemic disturbance is variable but sweating and pallor are common. The absence of significant fever helps to distinguish perforated ulcer from other common causes of an acute abdomen.

*The initial severe symptoms are often followed within a few hours by relief of pain and a general improvement only to be followed by sudden relapse and shock*.

Perforated peptic ulcer may occasionally be confused with other acute intra-abdominal conditions and more rarely with intrathoracic disease.

Suspicion of perforation demands admission to hospital where diagnosis will be confirmed by an erect X-ray of the abdomen and chest which shows free gas under the diaphragm.

If there is likely to be any delay and the patient is in severe pain, opiate analgesia should be considered. Alternative non opiate analgesia will be necessary if there is additional chronic respiratory disease.

## PENETRATION

Penetration occurs when an ulcer extends through the wall of the stomach or duodenum, but is prevented from perforating into the peritoneal cavity by other structures. The organ most commonly penetrated by a duodenal ulcer is the pancreas. This is characteristic of an ulcer of the posterior wall. It gives rise to radiation of pain to the back, which is more persistent and less readily relieved by standard medical management.

42

Less commonly, an ulcer may erode into the liver or biliary system. Even more unusual is the formation of a fistula between the colon and either a duodenal or gastric ulcer. This leads to bacterial proliferation in the small intestine which, in turn, causes diarrhoea and steatorrhoea.

Nevertheless, many cases of penetration cause remarkably few additional symptoms, the complication only being recognized when the patient ultimately comes to surgery.

## PYLORIC STENOSIS

The incidence of pyloric stenosis is decreasing. This probably reflects a change in the natural history of the disease but it also seems likely that the decline has been accelerated by more effective medical treatment.

Mechanical obstruction of the pyloric channel, when due to peptic ulcer, results from a combination of active inflammation and fibrosis. Nearly 60% of patients presenting with the condition have a duodenal ulcer, whereas benign gastric ulcer is a rare cause. *It should be remembered that in more than one third of cases pyloric stenosis is due to gastric carcinoma.*

The characteristic feature of pyloric stenosis is the regular vomiting of large quantities of gastric contents. The vomitus contains food eaten hours before or even from the previous day. Other symptoms include those of gastro-oesophageal reflux and upper abdominal fullness, relief from which is obtained by induced vomiting. If the condition remains untreated dehydration, metabolic alkalosis, hypokalaemia and negative nitrogen balance ensue.

Vigorous palpation over the stomach will produce a succussion splash and gastric peristalsis may be visible. Diagnosis is confirmed by aspiration of more than 200 ml of gastric fluid after an overnight fast. A barium meal reveals a greatly enlarged and slowly emptying stomach. Distinction between gastric carcinoma and duodenal ulcer can usually be made by radiology, but endoscopy may be necessary if diagnosis is not clear.

The patients must be admitted to hospital. Gastric aspiration will be necessary in the majority of cases to prevent persistent vomiting. Dehydration and metabolic disturbance will be treated with an appropriate intravenous regime and if there is evidence of malnutrition parenteral feeding may also be given.

Because acute inflammation is a major component of the pyloric obstruction, bed rest and aspiration will often relieve the condition. A reduction in the volume of gastric aspirate is a good indication of initial success. An H₂-antagonist may then be given in an attempt to further reduce inflammation. In many instances this will enable the patient to take nutrition orally.

This provides an opportunity to improve the patient's general condition and time to assess whether surgical or medical management is the more appropriate.

When fibrosis is a major component of the pyloric obstruction surgery will be necessary. Truncal vagotomy with a pyloroplasty or gastrojejunostomy are the most commonly performed operations, but success has recently been claimed for proximal gastric vagotomy, combined with either duodenotomy or digital dilatation of the stenosis.

## POINTS TO REMEMBER

Physical signs may underestimate blood loss

Pulse rate greater than 100 per minute, systolic blood pressure below 100 mmHg or diastolic pressure below 65 mmHg indicate need for urgent transfusion

If pulse and blood pressure are normal in recumbent position repeat with patient sitting or standing

All patients with haematemesis should be admitted urgently to hospital

Similarly patients with continuing melaena require urgent admission

Initial severe symptoms of perforation are often followed by relief of pain and a general improvement only to be followed by sudden relapse and shock

Regular vomiting of large volumes may indicate pyloric stenosis

# 6
# Surgical Management of Peptic Ulcer

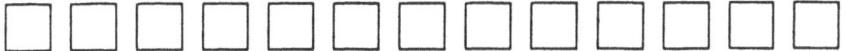

In the great majority of cases surgery, in contrast to medical therapy, provides a cure for both duodenal and gastric ulcers. Despite this, the number of operations for peptic ulcer has declined during the past decade. This reduction has undoubtedly been accelerated in recent years by cimetidine and ranitidine but other probable reasons are the falling incidence of ulcer disease and the increased acceptance by physicians and surgeons that a significant proportion of patients are dissatisfied with the result of their operation.

## TYPES OF OPERATION

All operations that are undertaken for peptic ulcer aim to reduce gastric acid secretion. This can be achieved by resection of a variable portion of the stomach or section of the vagus nerve.

The most commonly performed operations are illustrated in Figures 6.1–6.5.

## DUODENAL ULCER

### Selection of patients for surgery

The proportion of patients with duodenal ulcer requiring surgery is probably less than one in ten.

Failure of medical management constitutes approximately 50% of patients coming to operation. Within this group are those who:

- continue to have severe symptoms from an ulcer that fails to heal after an extended full dose course of an ulcer healing drug or a combination of two preparations,

- repeatedly relapse within a few weeks of stopping a healing course of treatment, particularly if they decide against maintenance treatment,

- frequently relapse whilst on a maintenance regime,

- have a long history of frequent severe exacerbations and do not wish to persist with medical therapy.

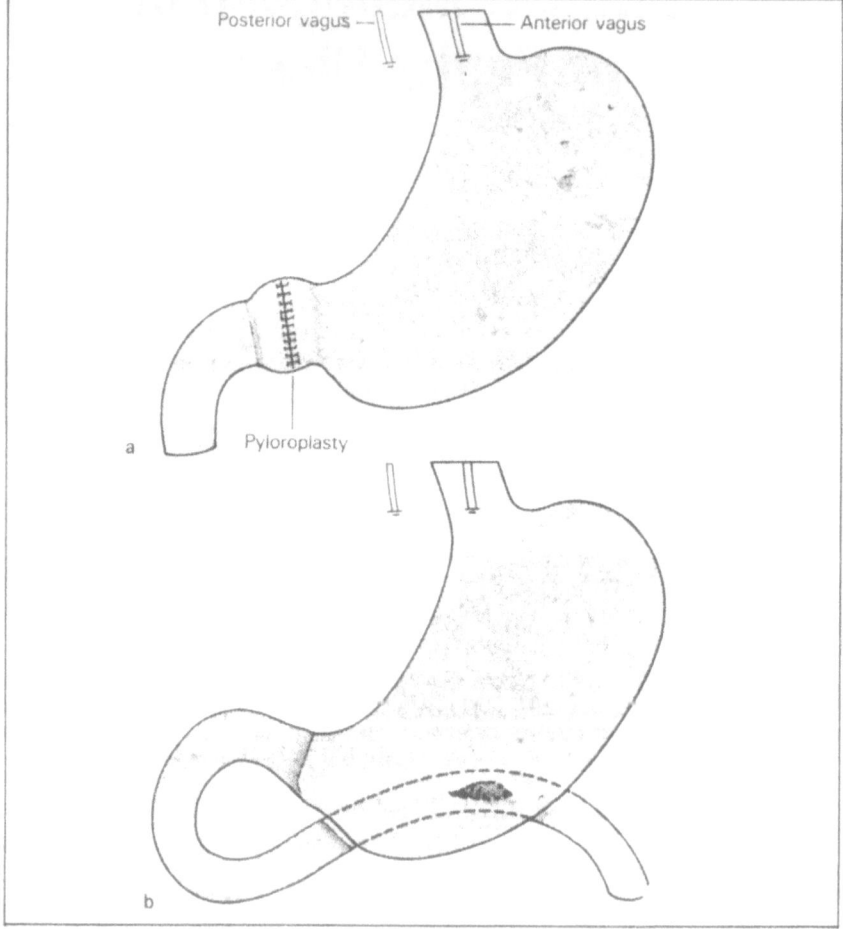

**Figure 6.1** Truncal vagotomy leads to gastric stasis and so is combined with a drainage procedure, most commonly pyloroplasty (**a**). In the presence of duodenal scarring and deformity, however, a gastrojejunostomy (**b**) is less hazardous

Additional factors that sway a decision towards surgery are a past history of bleeding, particularly if this has occurred more than once, and previous perforation.

The remaining 50% of patients receiving definitive surgery have their operation because of complications such as haemorrhage, pyloric stenosis or perforation.

## Selection of operation

The overriding consideration in deciding on which operation should be performed for duodenal ulcer must be its mortality. However, an operation with a low mortality is of limited use if it does not cure the presenting disease or leaves the patient with symptoms that are worse than those of the ulcer itself. These include recurrent ulceration, diarrhoea, dumping, vomiting, gastric stasis and nutritional disturbance. It must also be remembered that if a second operation is necessary this will inevitably increase the overall mortality.

Global assessment and patient satisfaction are difficult to measure but Visick grading is probably the best means of attempting this. Use of this method over long follow-up period has not yet shown that a particular operation is superior to the others.

## Mortality

There have been numerous studies involving large numbers of patients that show proximal gastric vagotomy has a mortality of less than 0.5%. This compares with a 1.6% mortality reported for vagotomy with antrectomy, and 2–6% for partial gastrectomy.

## Recurrent ulcer

Cumulative data from Europe and the USA show that the recurrence of ulcer after proximal gastric vagotomy is about 10%; following vagotomy and drainage it is approximately 8%, whereas the rate after vagotomy and antrectomy is only 1.4%. The reason for recurrence is not clear, but it is usually attributed to faulty tehnique with failure to perform an adequate vagotomy. The recurrence rate for proximal gastric vagotomy may be artificially low because the procedure is relatively new and it is generally accepted that recurrence of ulceration may occur many years after surgery.

Gastrojejunostomy alone is associated with a very high rate of recurrence, but it was recently proposed as a safe and simple procedure if limited to

47

GASTROENTEROLOGY

duodenal ulcer patients with a low acid output. Bilroth I gastrectomy is also complicated by very frequent ulcer recurrence and cannot be advocated for the treatment of duodenal ulcer. By contract Polya gastrectomy is followed by a recurrence rate of less than 2%.

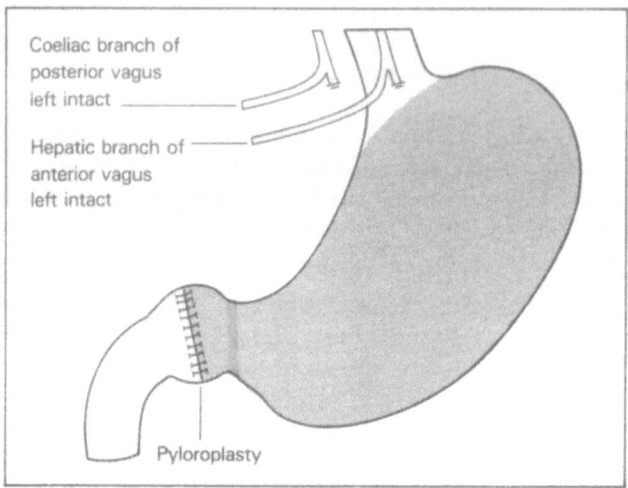

**Figure 6.2** Selective vagotomy and pyloroplasty. Selective cutting of the vagal nerve does not obviate the need for a drainage procedure, and pyloroplasty or jejunostomy is still necessary

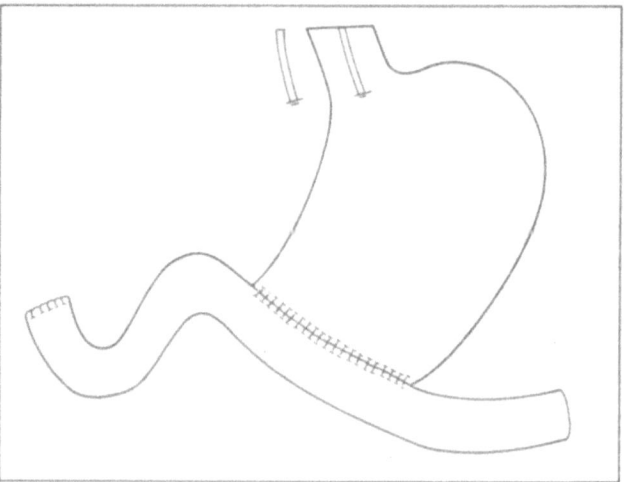

**Figure 6.3** Vagotomy and antrectomy aims to reduce acid secretion by removing both gastrin-secreting tissue and the neural stimulation of the parietal cells

48

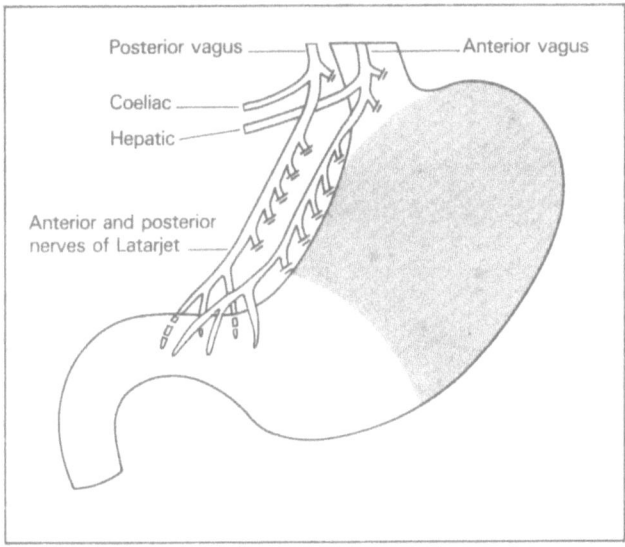

**Figure 6.4**  Proximal gastric vagotomy. This technique of highly selective vagotomy leaves the motility of the antrum and pylorus unaffected, so that a drainage procedure is not required

## Diarrhoea

Diarrhoea in the early postoperative period is common after many types of gastric surgery. It tends to improve with time but some patients continue to have sudden attacks of diarrhoea which can disable them for many years. The problem is equally bad following truncal vagotomy and drainage procedure or truncal vagotomy and antrectomy. In contrast it is a relatively minor problem after selective vagotomy and pyloroplasty, proximal gastric vagotomy without pyloroplasty or partial gastrectomy.

## Dumping

As with diarrhoea, dumping tends to be most severe in the first few months after the operation but a long term follow-up study in Leeds showed that it could still be a significant problem 5–8 years later. It is a complication of both partial gastrectomy and truncal vagotomy with drainage but the incidence is very low after proximal gastric vagotomy.

Other problems such as *bilious vomiting* and *gastric stasis* are also considerably less common after proximal gastric vagotomy than the other operations under discussion.

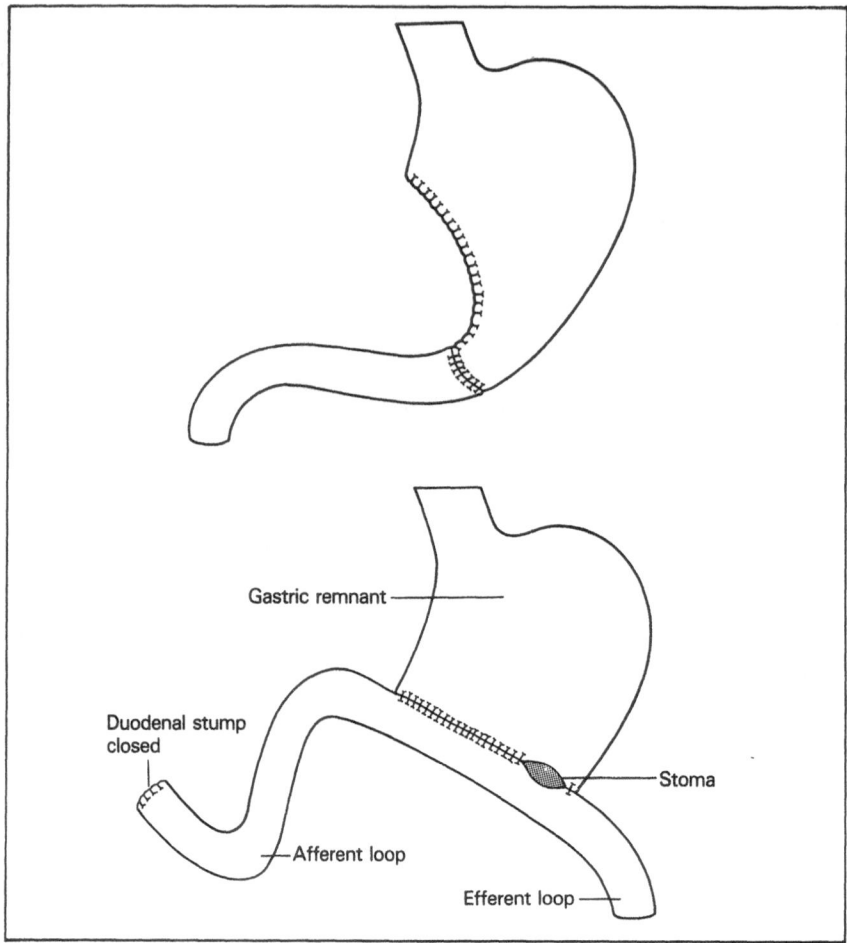

**Figure 6.5** In partial gastrectomy approximately two-thirds of the distal stomach is resected. The remnant is then anastomosed either (**a**) to the duodenum (Bilroth I gastrectomy) or (**b**) to the jejunum (Bilroth II gastrectomy)

## Nutritional disturbance

### *Iron deficiency anaemia*

This occurs in approximately 25% of patients 5 years after partial gastrectomy and an incidence of 50% has been noted in longer follow-up studies. Vagotomy and gastrojejunostomy are also complicated by microcytic anaemia, but the onset tends to be later. In contrast vagotomy and pyloroplasty and proximal gastric vagotomy do not predispose to iron deficiency.

## Megalobastic anaemia

Megaloblastic anaemia due to $B_{12}$ malabsorption is seen many years after partial gastrectomy in about 2% of patients but does not appear to complicate vagotomy.

## Osteomalacia

Osteomalacia after partial gastrectomy is an even rarer late complication, appearing in approximately 1%.

## Weight loss

Failure to regain a normal weight after surgery is seen in about half of those who have partial gastrectomy, in a third of those treated by vagotomy with gastroenterostomy and in less than 10% of patients undergoing vagotomy and pyloroplasty.

## Conclusion

In summary, it is likely that proximal gastric vagotomy will become increasingly popular as the operation of first choice in the treatment of duodenal ulcer because of the very low mortality and incidence of unwanted effects. But its major disadvantage is the relatively high rate of recurrent ulceration and if with longer periods of follow-up this increases still further, reappraisal will be necessary.

## GASTRIC ULCER

### Selection of patients for surgery

The indications for surgery in gastric ulcer are the same as those for duodenal ulcer, namely, failure of medical management and the occurrence of complications. In practice the operation is frequently offered earlier than in duodenal ulcer because complications such as bleeding and perforation have a worse prognosis. Furthermore, even when multiple biopsies show no evidence of cancer there is always the suspicion that a persisting gastric ulcer may be malignant.

### Selection of operation

The selection of the operation for gastric ulcer is less controversial than for duodenal ulcer. Whichever operation is performed, approximately 80% will have a satisfactory result.

Most experience has been with gastrectomy, usually a Bilroth I procedure. The mortality is in the order of 1–2% and the recurrence rate is about 2%. Recurrence after gastrectomy is lowest (less than 1%) when the original ulcer is on the lesser curve or in the body of the stomach. It is considerably higher (approximately 10%) in those with pyloric ulcers and when a gastric ulcer is accompanied by a duodenal ulcer. This group tends to secrete greater quantities of acid and because of this gastrectomy is frequently combined with vagotomy which reduces the recurrence rate to less than 5%.

Truncal vagotomy with drainage and proximal gastric vagotomy have been compared with Bilroth I gastrectomy. The recurrence rate after the former two procedures is approximately twice that found after gastrectomy. When a gastrectomy is not performed it is usual practice to resect the ulcer so that misdiagnosis of gastric cancer is avoided.

In summary, Bilroth I gastrectomy is the procedure of choice for most patients with gastric ulcer but this should probably be combined with a vagotomy in those who have pyloric or associated duodenal ulceration. Future studies may show that this group would be treated adequately by vagotomy and drainage or even proximal gastric vagotomy, thereby avoiding the complications of gastric resection.

The other sequelae of surgery for gastric ulcer are the same as those that follow duodenal ulcer surgery.

## MANAGEMENT OF THE SEQUELAE OF GASTRIC SURGERY

### Recurrent ulceration

Recurrence of an ulcer is usually heralded by return of pain but bleeding or penetration are alternative presentations. Approximately 60% of these lesions heal on cimetidine but the majority will ultimately require further surgery. In the past this has been accompanied by a mortality considerably greater than that for a first operation. However, two recently published series had a relatively low re-operation mortality of between 1 and 2%. Recurrence after gastrectomy requires the addition of vagotomy and following proximal gastric vagotomy or vagotomy and drainage, a revagotomy and antrectomy are usually performed.

### Diarrhoea

Diarrhoea is usually due to a combination of rapid gastric emptying and disturbance of bowel motility because of vagotomy. The tendency to diarrhoea improves with time but when the problem persists management is difficult because attacks are sporadic. However, when bouts are more prolonged prophylactic codeine phosphate or loperamide may prove helpful.

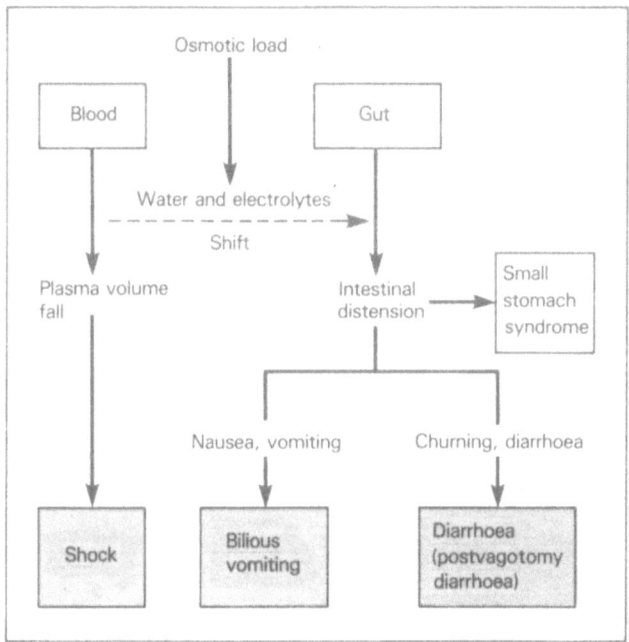

**Figure 6.6** Mechanisms of dumping syndromes (from Hobsley, M. (1984). Disturbances of physiology after gastric surgery. In Lancaster-Smith, M. (ed.) *Peptic Ulcer*. (London: Update Publications))

## Dumping (Figure 6.6)

*Early dumping*, which comes on during a meal or up to 1 hour afterwards, is caused by rapid discharge of hypertonic gastric contents into the small intestine.

The symptoms – which include faintness, flushing, palpitation, sweating and nausea – have been attributed to hypovolaemia. This is contributed to by the osmotic attraction of vascular space fluid into the gut lumen, but it seems likely that vasoactive peptides released from the upper small bowel are also important.

As with diarrhoea the severity of the problem diminishes with time, but can also be lessened by taking small meals low in carbohydrate and without additional fluid. When possible, the patient should lie down at the first suggestion of an attack. Anticholinergics to slow gastric emptying are of limited value. Guar gum as used in diabetes may be worthy of trial. When the problem is severe and persistent it may be necessary to revise the operation or reverse a loop of jejunum.

*Late dumping* is due to hypoglycaemia which comes on up to 3 hours after a meal. The exact mechanism is not clear but is partly due to a rapid release of insulin in response to a sudden rise in blood sugar which results from rapid gastric emptying. It is also likely that gastric surgery disturbs the subtle coordinated release of other upper gastrointestinal hormones.

The carbohydrate content of meals should be kept to a minimum in the hope of reducing excessive insulin release but if symptoms do occur they can usually be arrested by taking a small quantity of sucrose or glucose.

## Bilious vomiting

Vomiting or regurgitation of large quantities of bile-stained secretions is commonest after Polya gastrectomy or gastrojejunostomy, but also occurs after pyloroplasty. If persistent it may be necessary to perform a 'biliary diversion' operation, but milder cases can usually be managed by metoclopramide soon after meals and hydrotalcite or aluminium hydroxide between meals.

## Nutritional disturbance

A subnormal weight is usually the result of inadequate intake because of anorexia, loss of taste, or sensation of fullness during meals. Reassurance that the problem is not progressive and encouragement to take more protein are all that is usually required. Only rarely does gastric surgery lead to a classical malabsorption syndrome. A blind loop syndrome should be considered in those with a Polya gastrectomy.

## Anaemia

The commonest cause of anaemia is iron deficiency due to malabsorption from the duodenum. *It may present at any time after surgery* and is most common in premenopausal women. The mechanisms include inadequate mixing of food with gastric acid, hypochlorhydria, rapid transit through the upper bowel and, in some instances, bypass of the duodenum.

*Patients who have undergone gastric surgery should have their haemoglobin checked annually*. If this is not feasible they should be given an annual 3-month course of oral iron or a single daily ferrous sulphate tablet indefinitely.

If the annual blood film shows macrocytosis the most likely cause will be vitamin $B_{12}$ deficiency due to inadequate intrinsic factor. Two monthly intramuscular injections of Neocytamen 1 mg is the appropriate treatment.

More rarely macrocytosis is due to folate deficiency which may result either from inadequate intake or malabsorption.

## Metabolic bone disease

Osteomalacia is probably the major component of bone disease after gastrectomy, but osteoporosis is a contributory factor. It is rare, occurring in less than 1% of men and about 4% of women. The characteristic symptoms are bone pain and muscle weakness. There may be reduced serum levels of calcium and phosphate but the commonest biochemical abnormality is a raised serum alkaline phosphatase. Further confirmation of the diagnosis is obtained by X-ray or more rarely by bone biopsy. Treatment is with vitamin D and calcium supplements.

# 7

# Gastrointestinal Bleeding

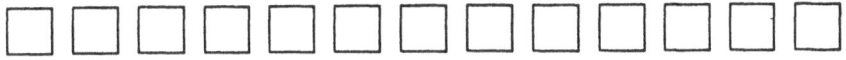

This can be subdivided into

(1)  acute upper gastrointestinal haemorrhage,

(2)  chronic or recurrent bleeding,

(3)  rectal bleeding.

Acute haemorrhage from the oesophagus, stomach and upper small intestine gives rise to haematemesis and/or melaena, whereas melaena alone is the result of bleeding from the lower small intestine or caecum. Bleeding from sites distal to the ascending colon presents as identifiable blood being passed per rectum. Chronic bleeding from the alimentary tract often causes no change in the faeces and presents most commonly as anaemia.

## ACUTE UPPER GASTROINTESTINAL HAEMORRHAGE

### Common causes

In Britain, bleeding from the upper gastrointestinal tract results in approximately 25 000 admissions to hospitals each year. Mortality lies between 5 and 10%. The commonest causes are duodenal ulcer (40%), while gastric ulcer and gastric erosions account for 15% each. Gastric cancer, oesophagitis and tears of the lower oesophagus each constitute 5%. Bleeding from oesophageal varices is relatively uncommon in Britain and accounts for approximately 3%. These percentages are approximate and are extracted from several studies over the past 25 years. Leiomyomas and acute stress ulcers following burns or shock are rare causes. No definite cause is found in approximately 10% of patients despite investigation (Figures 7.1 and 7.2).

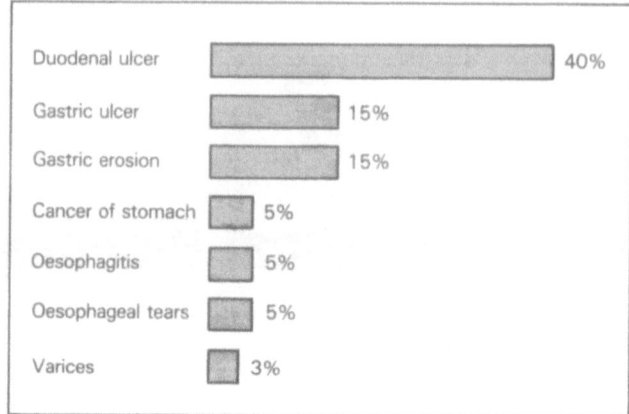

**Figure 7.1**   Causes of upper gastrointestinal bleeding in the UK (cumulative data 1955–80)

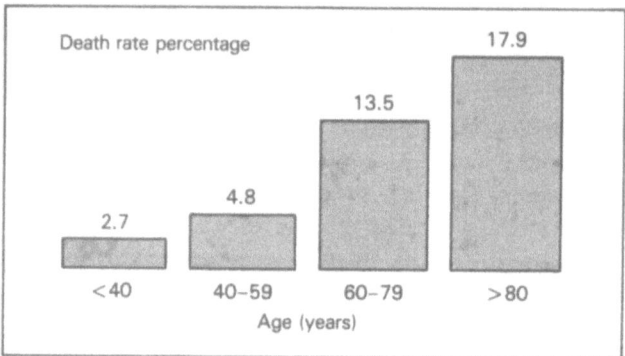

**Figure 7.2**   The effect of age on the death rate in patients admitted to the Radcliffe Infirmary, Oxford, with haematemesis and melaena from Schiller, K.F.R., Truelove, S.C. and Williams, D.G. (1970). *Br. Med. J.*, **2,** 7

## Assessment of severity

Haematemesis may consist of either fresh blood mixed with gastric contents, or changed blood in the form of 'coffee grounds'. However, blood discovered in the mouth may also have originated from the postnasal space or the respiratory tract. An accurate history is very important to try to differentiate the cause.

A patient's assessment of the amount of blood vomited is not usually helpful. Haematemesis may be accompanied by melaena but if help is sought immediately melaena may not always be present initially. Rectal examination is mandatory to confirm melaena. Melaena without haematemesis often indicates a less severe bleed. *All patients with haematemesis should be admitted to hospital. Similarly if melaena is fresh or has been present for 3 days or less, admission is required.* A longer history of intermittent melaena in a patient who is not anaemic and is otherwise healthy does not necessarily require admission as long as early investigation can be arranged. Melaena may sometimes be confused with stools of patients taking iron- or bismuth-containing preparations as they both cause dark faeces. *Neither iron nor bismuth gives a positive occult blood test.*

Physical signs following gastrointestinal haemorrhage are frequently misleading and it is easy to underestimate the true blood loss. Pallor of the skin, a pulse rate of more than 100/min, a systolic blood pressure of less than 100 mmHg or a diastolic blood pressure of less than 65 mmHg all indicate the need for blood transfusion. If these measurements are taken with the patient lying down, hypovolaemia may not be detected. Thus, if normal, they should be repeated with the patient standing or sitting. A drop of pressure or rise in pulse rate are indications of a significant drop in blood volume. Estimation of the central venous pressure is an even more accurate means of assessing the degree of hypovolaemia. A haemoglobin concentration of less than 9 g/100 ml suggests severe haemorrhage. However, vasoconstriction can maintain a misleadingly high haemoglobin concentration, so normal levels do not exclude haemorrhage.

In most hospitals patients with haematemesis and melaena are admitted under the care of a physician, but surgical teams should be kept informed of the patient's progress since surgical intervention is often required.

### Clinical features

A history of previous peptic ulcer may be helpful although it does not prove that there is an existing ulcer or that it is the bleeding site. A significant proportion of patients who bleed from peptic ulcers have no history of dyspepsia. Aspirin and anti-inflammatory drugs cause gastrointestinal haemorrhage. The role of aspirin in this context has probably been overstated. A history of aspirin consumption in the previous 48 hours does not necessarily indicate that bleeding is due to gastric erosion, and evidence that steroids cause significant gastrointestinal haemorrhage is even more tenuous. Alcohol abuse should be considered in patients with peptic ulcer, gastric erosions, oesophageal varices and tears. In the latter case, which may not always be alcohol induced, haematemesis is usually preceded by vomiting without blood.

Although cutaneous signs of chronic liver disease, splenomegaly and ascites suggest the possibility of variceal bleeding, it is worth remembering that both peptic ulcer and gastric erosions are commonly associated with cirrhosis. Recent weight loss, anorexia or a mass in the epigastrium point to a diagnosis of stomach cancer. Carcinoma of the caecum may be identified by a mass in the right iliac fossa or a change of bowel habit and may give rise to melaena.

The great majority of patients with acute gastrointestinal haemorrhage have a local lesion in the gut. The remaining small proportion is accounted for by diseases such as bleeding diatheses, leukaemia, polyarteritis nodosa, Henoch–Schönlein purpura and chronic renal failure. These are usually evident after simple routine investigation. *The site of bleeding can be identified in more than 95% of cases by endoscopy if performed within 24 hours of the haemorrhage.*

## CHRONIC OR RECURRENT BLEEDING

Recurrent haematemeses are uncommon except in the case of a patient with oesophageal varices in whom sclerosant therapy has not been adopted or completed. Such recurrences frequently occur in hospital. Other causes of severe acute bleeding have usually been diagnosed endoscopically and promptly treated.

In contrast, chronic blood loss of small quantities from the oesophagus, stomach, small intestine and caecum most commonly presents as iron deficiency anaemia and occasionally as melaena. Haemorrhage from more distal sites usually presents as identifiable blood per rectum and is discussed below (under Rectal Bleeding). All conditions which present with acute bleeding can also cause chronic blood loss. Attention to previously discussed clinical features, appropriate barium studies and endoscopy will reveal the site in the majority of cases. When melaena is not obvious, occult blood may be found if stools are examined, confirming alimentary tract blood loss. The following are less common causes of chronic gastrointestinal bleeding.

(1) *Hereditary haemorrhage telangectasia.* This is inherited by autosomal dominance so usually there is a family history. Obvious lesions are found on the lips and buccal mucosa, around the nostrils and under the nails.

(2) *Lymphoma of the gut.* This must always be considered when routine investigations have failed to demonstrate a cause. Abdominal masses, peripheral lymphadenopathy, splenomegaly and constitutional disturbance may be present also.

(3) *Polyposis* of the small intestine is a rare cause of recurrent blood loss. The Peutz–Jeghers syndrome consists of dark brown pigmentation of the lips and buccal mucosa, together with hamartomatous polyps in the small intestine. This is inherited by autosomal dominance so there is usually a family history.

(4) *Hookworm* infestation especially is a cause in the developing countries. Stool examination is diagnostic.

(5) *Intra-abdominal artificial arterial grafts* occasionally form a fistula with the gut. The commonest site is between the aorta and the third part of the duodenum. In this particular group of patients it is important to watch for this possibility as small bleeds usually precede a massive fatal haemorrhage.

Selective angiography of the mesenteric arteries is now used when routine barium studies and endoscopy have failed to demonstrate a lesion. If this procedure is conducted during a bleed, extravasation of the radio-opaque medium can be seen. When the patient is not bleeding, arteriography may show the typical pattern of a vascular tumour or angiodysplasia.

---

*Points to stress*

- Haematemesis indicates recent haemorrhage and the need for hospital admission

- In a patient with gastrointestinal bleeding, a postural drop in blood pressure and rise in pulse rate indicates hypovolaemia and the need for urgent blood replacement

- A normal haemoglobin does not exclude significant blood loss

---

## RECTAL BLEEDING

Rectal bleeding means the passage of identifiable blood per rectum as distinct from melaena stool. It is most likely due to blood loss from the colon and rectum. Occasionally brisk bleeding from the upper gastrointestinal tract can result in rectal bleeding. However, rectal bleeding is rarely heavy and does not usually necessitate urgent admission.

## Investigations

As discussed below, careful history taking and examination should obviate the need for unnecessary investigation. Thus patients who present with a small amount of blood on the stool or toilet paper should all have a digital examination. If no local anal cause can be found and treated they should be referred for sigmoidoscopy and further investigation in hospital.

## Common causes

### Haemorrhoids

Approximately 90% of rectal bleeding is accounted for by haemorrhoids. Blood is found on the stools and on the toilet paper. Patients rarely complain of pain unless there is thrombosis or a perianal haematoma after straining at stool. Occasionally fresh blood alone may be passed. First-degree piles are diagnosed by proctoscopy. Second-degree piles are obvious when the patient strains. Third-degree piles are prolapsed.

First- and minor second-degree piles are best treated by sclerosant injection. Larger second-degree piles require haemorrhoidectomy and/or manual dilation under anaesthesia. The majority of patients suffering with piles tend to be constipated and it is important to give them dietary advice and encourage regular bowel habits, preferably with the use of bulk purgatives to try to reduce the chance of recurrence.

### Anal fissure

Although an anal fissure may bleed, most patients present with pain during defaecation. Diagnosis is confirmed by gently parting the buttocks. It is usually impossible to undertake rectal examination at the patient's first consultation, owing to pain. Treatment consists in the first place of using an anaesthetic gel applied with an applicator or digitally and attention to avoiding constipation. An anal dilator with anaesthetic gel is the next step. In more severe cases surgical division of part of the internal anal sphincter may be necessary. Proctoscopy should be done when feasible to exclude carcinoma or inflammatory bowel disease.

### Polyps

Excluding anal disease, polyps of the large bowel are the next commonest cause of rectal bleeding (it is usually the only symptom). The patient should be referred forthwith. Diagnosis is confirmed by sigmoidoscopy and failing this, *double contrast* barium enema. Single contrast techniques do not give sufficient differentiation to find small polyps. It may be necessary for the flexible colonoscope to be used, when the lesions may be resected without resorting to laparotomy or colotomy. All adenomatous polyps are now removed, because of the risk of carcinomatous change.

## Large bowel cancer

The majority of large bowel cancers bleed, but bleeding may only be slight or occult. Severe bleeding is rare. The only symptom may be rectal bleeding but usually there is tenesmus, altered bowel habit and abdominal pain. Weight loss and anorexia, while they occur, do not have the same prevalence as in other cancers. Abdominal examination may reveal a mass. Digital examination of the rectum will demonstrate a high proportion of rectal carinomas and many in the sigmoid colon will be palpable extrinsically. Investigations are those used for polyps. The patient may be anaemic. Sixty per cent of all large bowel cancers can be diagnosed by sigmoidoscopy.

## Inflammatory bowel disease

Both ulcerative colitis and Crohn's disease may present with rectal bleeding, but in both it is usually accompanied by diarrhoea and in Crohn's disease by abdominal pain. The patient should be referred and investigation follows the same lines as for polyps and cancer.

## Diverticular disease

In developed countries, diverticula of the colon may be found in more than a third of the population over 60. Although diverticula do bleed either overtly or occultly, their relative commonness means an alternative cause should also be excluded. The most useful differentiating test is angiography during a phase of bleeding.

## Rarer causes

### Infection

Shigella and amoebic dysentry cause rectal bleeding but both are unusual in the British Isles.

Salmonella and Campylobacter can affect the large intestine. The bleeding is accompanied by diarrhoea and the illness is usually brief.

## Ischaemia

Ischaemia of the colon may lead to rectal bleeding. Symptoms consist of pain, guarding, pyrexia and systemic disturbance. There is usually evidence of cardiovascular disease and it is commonest in the elderly. Ischaemia may cause infarction of the bowel necessitating resection. Alternatively there may be return to normal bowel function in a few days. Ischaemic strictures may develop, presenting as obstruction. Some may require surgical intervention but many resolve over weeks or months.

## Angiodysplasia

Angiodysplasia is a recently recognized vascular abnormality of the gut mucosa. It may give rise to melaena or rectal bleeding. It is thought to be a degenerative disorder and thus is most common in the elderly. The usual site is the right colon. Diagnosis is best confirmed by angiography.

Cautery via the colonoscope is often possible. Extensive lesions may require resection.

## Massive rectal bleeding

This is, as previously mentioned, an uncommon event. The causes in adults are: diverticular disease, inflammatory bowel disease, colorectal tumours and angiodysplasia. A Meckel's diverticulum should be considered in young adults and adolescents. Admission to hospital is imperative.

# 8

# Acute Abdominal Pain

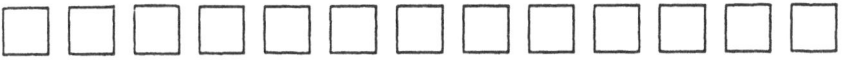

Acute abdominal pain is one of the commonest reasons for requesting an emergency hospital admission.

Patients with this problem require rapid assessment. A thorough history as outlined below and a full general examination are essential.

### HISTORY

This should be elicited preferably from the patient, but when he or she is too distressed much valuable information can be obtained from relatives or companions.

### Site

The 'typical' sites are illustrated in Figure 8.1, but it must be emphasized that there may be much variation.

### Onset

The onset is typically *sudden* in:

- perforation of a viscus
  rupture of an aortic aneurysm
  infarction of bowel

65

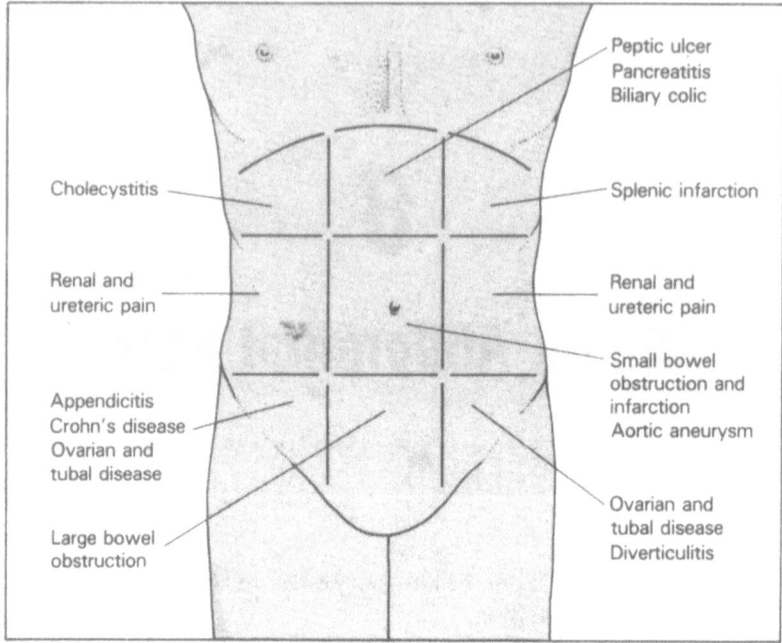

Peptic ulcer
Pancreatitis
Biliary colic

Cholecystitis

Splenic infarction

Renal and
ureteric pain

Renal and
ureteric pain

Small bowel
obstruction and
infarction
Aortic aneurysm

Appendicitis
Crohn's disease
Ovarian and
tubal disease

Ovarian and
tubal disease
Diverticulitis

Large bowel
obstruction

**Figure 8.1** 'Typical' sites of abdominal pain

It tends to be *more gradual* when inflammation is the cause, as in:

- appendicitis
  cholecystitis
  pancreatitis
  diverticulitis
  urinary tract inflammation
  salpingitis
  gastroenteritis

Severity may *increase progressively* over a few hours as with biliary colic.

## Type

The pain of *renal colic* is characterized by severe spasm superimposed on a more constant pain in a very restless patient.

*Biliary colic* is a misnomer because typically there are no spasms but rather a steadily increasing pain which crescendoes over 1–3 hours.

*Bowel colic* is usually punctuated by pain-free periods.

Patients who survive a *ruptured aortic aneurysm* describe an initial tearing pain.

*Intestinal infarction* is accompanied by very severe localized pain often with little abdominal tenderness.

## Duration

The evolution of the pain after admission may be helpful in assisting diagnosis.

Obvious perforation or infarction tends to be dealt with by immediate surgery and so the pain is shortlived. Pain of lesser severity which is frequently treated more conservatively is usually the result of inflammation or obstruction.

## Relieving or aggravating factors

Typically a patient with peritonitis from any cause sits or lies completely still because movement aggravates the pain. By contrast, patients with colic find it impossible to stay still.

## Additional features

Previous *dyspepsia* in a patient with peritonism would suggest perforation of an ulcer as the cause.

*Anorexia and weight loss* might indicate an alimentary tract carcinoma which may have perforated or caused obstruction.

*Bleeding per rectum* is suggestive of carcinoma, diverticulitis, bowel infarction or acute inflammatory bowel disease.

*Profuse diarrhoea* is likely to indicate acute gastroenteritis. It may be possible to identify potential causes such as the ingestion during the previous 72 hours of:

- previously frozen food
- inadequately cooked chicken
- cold meats or pies

A history of progressive *constipation* may precede intestinal obstruction due to carcinoma or diverticulitis.

*Alcohol* abuse might be the cause of an irritant gastritis or acute pancreatitis.

Similarly *drugs* – especially the non-steroidal anti-inflammatory agents – may cause severe abdominal pain, usually due to gastric irritation.

A *missed period* raises the possibility of an ectopic pregnancy, and a *vaginal discharge* salpingitis.

*Dysuria and haematuria* point to a urinary tract pathology.

## EXAMINATION

### General

A thorough general examination is essential, including measurement of temperature, pulse and blood pressure.

The *skin* and *sclera* may be *icteric*, indicating probable hepatobiliary or pancreatic disease.

*Ketoacidosis* which is often accompanied by acute abdominal pain can be identified by the characteristic *foetor*.

### Cardiorespiratory

Signs of *heart failure* may be found following *myocardial infarction* which occasionally confusingly causes severe upper abdominal pain. Patients with atrial fibrillation are likely candidates for mesenteric arterial embolization.

In the respiratory system *signs of lobar pneumonia* should be specifically searched for.

### Abdomen

*Scars of previous surgery* raise the possibility of a recurrent pathology or intestinal obstruction due to adhesions.

There may be obvious *distension* in patients with bowel obstruction or from ascites in those with malignant disease.

Localized *tenderness and guarding* usually indicate inflammatory disease, and rigidity generalized peritonitis.

*Non-tender masses* point to an underlying malignancy, whereas obvious *tenderness over a mass* is usually indicative of inflammatory disease such as appendicitis, cholecystitis, diverticulitis, Crohn's disease or salpingitis. An aortic aneurysm is characterized by expansile pulsation.

Kidney pathology will be missed if the *renal angles* are not specifically examined.

*Rectal examination* may identify a rectrocaecal appendicitis or diverticulitis of the sigmoid colon and help to localize the site of pathology to the bladder, prostate or female reproductive organs.

*Vaginal examination* is essential in the presence of a vaginal discharge and when gynaecological disease is suspected.

*Auscultation* may reveal the exaggerated bowel sounds of intestinal obstruction or their absence in paralytic ileus due to peritoneal irritation. With an aortic aneurysm a bruit may be audible.

The *male external genitalia* must be examined to exclude torsion of the testis and epididymo-orchitis which often give rise to severe pain referred to the abdomen.

Finally the *inguinal areas* must be inspected and palpated for enlarged lymph nodes and herniae.

## DISCRIMINATING FEATURES

Information gained in the above way will suggest likely provisional diagnoses and enable a referral to be made to the appropriate hospital department.

The following are helpful discriminating features of those abdominal diseases that commonly cause acute pain.

### Appendicitis

Features are:

    initial central abdominal pain
    movement of pain to right iliac fossa
    mild to moderate pyrexia
    tenderness and guarding in right iliac fossa
    tenderness to the right on rectal examination

*Beware*
(1) the obese patient in whom adequate abdominal examination may be difficult.
(2) pregnancy, because the appendix may be displaced into the right hypochondrium.

### Mesenteric adenitis

This is most common in children but should be considered in adolescents and young adults.

Look for:
    features of upper respiratory tract infection
    pyrexia

69

lower abdominal tenderness and guarding

It is often impossible to distinguish preoperatively from appendicitis.

## Diverticulitis

This is unusual in under-60 age group.

Features are:

pyrexia and malaise
lower abdominal pain and guarding, left more commonly than right
mass in pouch of Douglas on rectal examination
frequency of micturition due to spread of infection to bladder

Many patients can be treated successfully at home with a liquid diet and broad spectrum antibiosis. *Perforation* causes severe systemic disturbance and peritonism.

## Acute pancreatitis

Features are as follows:

the predominant symptom is upper abdominal pain radiating to the back
nausea and vomiting are very common
systemic disturbance varies from mild pyrexia to profound shock
there is guarding or even rigidity in severe cases
in fulminant cases bruising around the umbilicus and in the flanks may be
    seen
there may be a history of gallstones or alcohol abuse
admission to hospital is advisable
diagnosis can usually be confirmed by finding a greatly elevated serum
    amylase level during the acute phase
mild jaundice is common
pain that persists for more than a week may indicate a pseudocyst or
    abscess

## Gastroenteritis

Features are as follows:

pain is usually overshadowed by vomiting and or diarrhoea
occasionally pain predominates, especially in *Campylobacter* infection
associated malaise is often profound and accompanied by variable fever

## Gall bladder disease

### Biliary colic

Features are:

sudden onset
most intense in the epigastrium
unremitting pain which crescendos within 3 hours
vomiting is common but gives no relief
tenderness in upper abdomen
discomfort in upper abdomen for several days after acute episode

Need for potent analgesia usually requires admission to hospital.

### Acute cholecystitis

Features are:

possible progress from typical episode of biliary colic
increasingly severe pain mainly in right hypochondrium
persists up to 24–48 hours
radiation to back or subscapular region
pyrexia
tenderness along right costal margin
despite treatment with potent analgesics and broad spectrum antibiotics
  tenderness persists for many days.
mild jaundice and bile in the urine are commonly found

## Perforated peptic ulcer

Features are:

sudden severe epigastric pain is the presenting symptom
examination at this stage reveals board like rigidity and absent bowel
  sounds
But if delayed classical peritonism may be absent
rapid admission to hospital should be arranged where the diagnosis will be
  confirmed by the finding on X-ray of gas under the diaphragm
there is not always a history of dyspepsia

## Intestinal obstruction

Features are as follows:

large bowel obstruction often causes relatively little pain and may progress insidiously

small bowel obstruction tends to occur more suddenly and is frequently more painful

the abdomen is obviously distended and resonant to percussion

bowel sounds are often exaggerated and peristalsis may be visible

vomiting is not invariable and may occur very late in large bowel obstruction.

The common causes of intestinal obstruction are:

(1)   carcinoma of the large bowel

(2)   diverticular disease

(3)   peritoneal adhesions

(4)   hernias

Diagnosis is confirmed following admission to hospital by the finding of fluid levels in the bowel on the erect abdominal X-ray.

### Salpingitis

Features are:

suprapubic pain and tenderness
vaginal discharge
pain on palpating the cervix
confirmation is by laparoscopy or laparotomy

### Ectopic pregnancy

Features are:

a missed period
lower abdominal tenderness
a mass in the pouch of Douglas
vaginal bleeding may occur
if bleeding is massive, signs of shock and peritonism will predominate

### Ruptured aortic aneurysm

Features are:

possible preceding history of abdominal or back pain
often history or signs of peripheral vascular disease

a phase of hypotension is common, often with collapse
the aneurysm may be palpable and a bruit audible in the abdomen

*Immediate admission for emergency surgery is vital.*

## Bowel ischaemia

Features are:

sudden onset of severe pain and tenderness (the site is dependent upon whether the superior or inferior mesenteric is involved).
cause is often embolic due to atrial fibrillation
bloody diarrhoea or frank blood loss per rectum may be found
if ischaemic is extensive shock and severe peritonism will be present

## Renal colic

Features are:

pain is predominantly in the flank or back
radiation to groin or testicle is common
often accompanied by urge to micturate
there may be macroscopic or microscopic blood loss per urethram

## Pyelonephritis

Features are:

pain is again predominantly felt in the renal angles and tenderness is found on palpation
fever and even rigors are common
dysuria when present is virtually diagnostic

## Abdominal pain in other diseases

Rarely abdominal pain may be a predominant feature of disease outside the abdomen or of a more generalized nature. The commonest causes are:

(1) lobar pneumonia
(2) myocardial infarction
(3) pericarditis
(4) diabetic ketoacidosis
(5) Henoch–Schönlein purpura

*These conditions should be considered whenever examination of the abdomen fails to reveal tenderness, guarding or rigidity.*

73

# 9

# Chronic Abdominal Pain

Recurrent abdominal pain is a common cause for seeking a consultant opinion but much useful information can be obtained by the general practitioner and in many instances successful management instituted.

It is important to note the following features of the pain or discomfort.

(1)  nature
(2)  severity
(3)  frequency
(4)  duration
(5)  site and radiation
(6)  precipitating and relieving factors

Abdominal pains are often related to eating and drinking. The commonest causes frequently associated with meals are:

peptic ulcer
the irritable bowel syndrome
gastric carcinoma
oesophagitis

Rare causes of postprandial pain are:

mesenteric angina
Crohn's disease
pancreatic disease

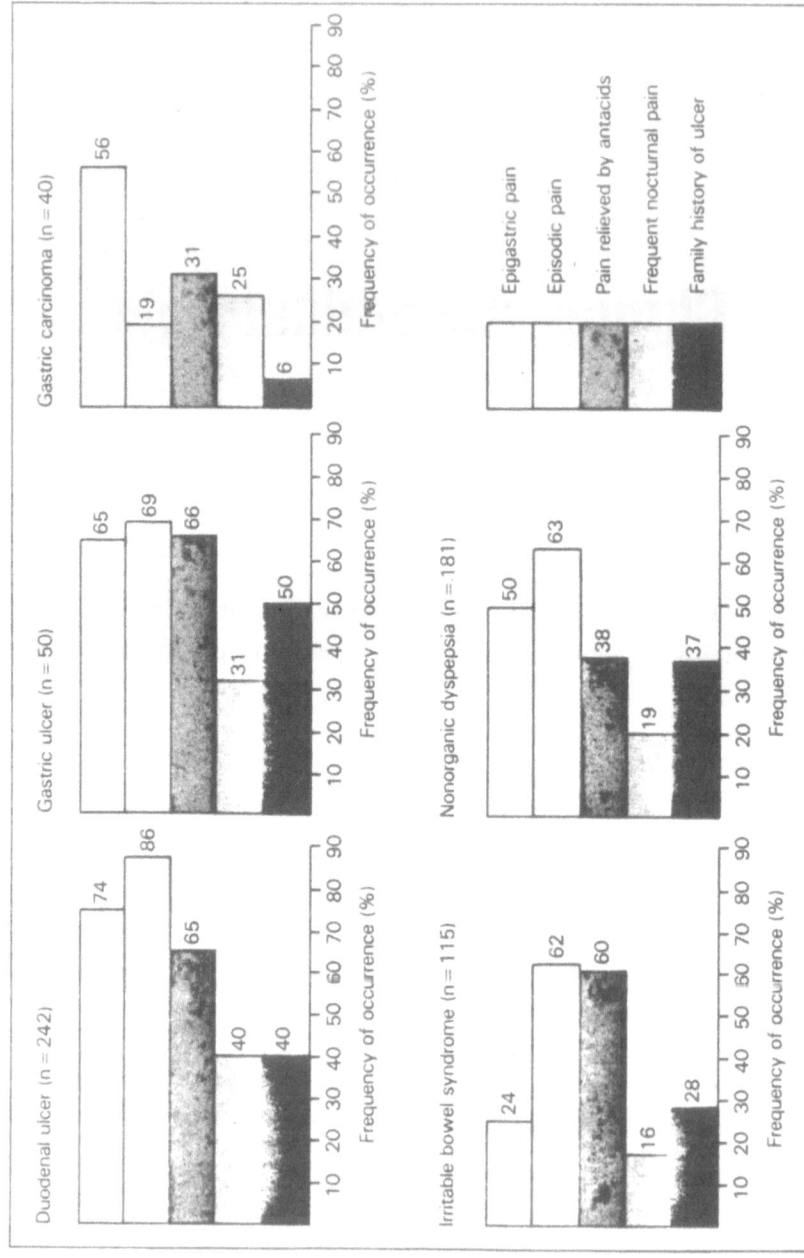

**Figure 9.1** Frequency of occurrence (%) of some symptoms in different 'dyspeptic' conditions (from Crean, G.P. (1984). Symptomatic diagnosis of dyspepsia. In Lancaster-Smith, M. (ed.) *Peptic Ulcer*. (London: Update Publications))

Pain inconsistently associated with mealtimes may be due to:

gastritis
aerophagy
psychological 'stress'

*Gallbladder pain has no consistent association with food.*


## DISCRIMINATORY FEATURES

Helpful discriminatory features of diseases that commonly cause chronic or recurrent abdominal pain are listed below.


### Peptic ulcer

Features are:

pain well localized, usually to the epigastrium, more rarely to the hypochondria
radiation retrosternally or to the back
attacks limited to a few hours
relief by vomiting or taking antacids
described as pain not discomfort
bouts last 1–2 weeks
remissions often last for months
nocturnal incidence common
tenderness in epigastrium is usually the only sign


### Gastric carcinoma

Features are:

pain usually epigastric
pain lacks periodicity and remissions do not occur
'fullness' after small amounts of food
anorexia and weight loss
abdominal mass may be palpable


### Irritable bowel syndrome

Features are:

often poorly localized discomfort rather than pain sometimes precipitated by meals

may be attacks of severe colic in lower abdomen eased or precipitated by
    defaecation
alternating frequency of defaecation and constipation
morning frequency of defaecation or passage of loose stool
nausea without vomiting

## Mesenteric angina

Features are:

severe central abdominal pain precipitated by meals
usually elderly patients with peripheral vascular disease or myocardial
    ischaemia

## Pancreatic disease

Features are:

both chronic or relapsing pancreatitis and carcinoma of the pancreas may
    cause recurrent or chronic abdominal pain
the site is epigastric with radiation to the back
it is a boring deep aching pain
food and alcohol are common precipitating factors
each attack lasts several hours
leaning forward or lying prone eases pain
with pancreatic cancer the pain eventually becomes continuous and is
    accompanied by anorexia
epigastric tenderness is often the only sign, but a mass may be palpable
    due to carcinoma or pseudocyst
there may be features of diabetes and malabsorption
mild jaundice and bilirubinuria are common

## Crohn's disease

Features are:

recurrent abdominal pain for years prior to presentation or diagnosis is
    very common
associated diarrhoea frequently occurs but is not invariable
features of malabsorption sometimes predominate
recurrent incomplete obstruction may occur
an inflammatory mass is sometimes palpable

## Colorectal cancer

Features are:

vague abdominal discomfort often precedes more definite symptoms or signs
a mass palpable abdominally or rectally
anaemia
blood loss per rectum
anorexia
weight loss

## Diverticular disease

Features are:

narrowing of the bowel lumen due to recurrent diverticulitis may cause colic and constipation
obstruction is a relatively rare complication
diverticulitis causes more severe localized pain with guarding, usually in the left iliac fossa, accompanied by pyrexia
associated dysuria may occur owing to spread of infection to the bladder
rectal bleeding which is occasionally profuse is common

## Gastritis

Chronic gastritis causing epigastric pain and discomfort may be due to:

drugs, especially non-steroidal anti-inflammatory agents
alcohol abuse
gastric surgery

## Aerophagy

Aerophagy causes distension of the stomach leading to pain and discomfort in the upper abdomen. It is particularly common in:
rapid eaters
heartburn sufferers
anxiety
severe psychiatric disturbance
Belching and flatus passed rectally are associated symptoms.

## 'Stress' dyspepsia

Features are:

pain is *not* well localized
it is seldom nocturnal
it is not consistently relieved by antacids or related to meals
non-gastrointestinal symptoms are common and include;
  headache
  lethargy
  depression
Management includes removal of stressful factors and treatment of depression

## Gall bladder disease

The symptoms and signs of gallbladder disease have been described in Chapter 8, 'Acute Abdominal Pain'.

Pain from gallbladder disease is rarely recurrent because severity demands urgent investigation and treatment.

*Gallbladder disease is not a cause of vague right hypochondrial pain or discomfort nor is it a cause of so-called flatulent dyspesia.*

## Hepatic pain

Persistent discomfort or pain in the right hypochondrium may be due to congestion of the liver in cardiac failure or expansion from secondary carcinoma.

## Renal pain

Kidney carcinoma or hydronephrosis can give rise to chronic pain in the flank. The urine should be examined for frank or microscopic haematuria.

## Musculoskeletal pain

Features are:

compression of thoracic or lumbar nerve roots can cause abdominal pain
accompanying back pain is usual and is frequently exacerbated or relieved
  by changes in posture
X-rays of the thoracic spine often show degenerative disease or a prolapsed disc

## Management

It is obviously impractical to investigate every patient who presents at the surgery with abdominal pain or discomfort.

The following is suggested as an approach to the problem.

(1)  When peptic ulcer seems to be the likely diagnosis on clinical evidence in a patient *under the age of 40*, give a trial of antacids and advise on diet and habits (see Chapter 4).

If relief is obtained no investigation is required.

By contrast, if relief is incomplete or symptoms rapidly return request barium meal.

On confirmation of peptic ulcer disease prescribe healing course of an appropriate drug (cimetidine, ranitidine, De-Nol, sucralfate).

(2)  In patients *over 40*, who are experiencing dyspeptic symptoms for the first time, investigation before treatment is advisable, because not to do so may delay the diagnosis of gastrointestinal cancer.

*Barium meal* is still the most readily accessible initial investigation available in general practice. It will detect about 80% of duodenal ulcers and the great majority of gastric cancers.

If the barium meal proves negative, but peptic disease or carcinoma are strongly suspected, *upper gastrointestinal endoscopy* should be arranged.

Lesions often missed by barium meal but detected at endoscopy include:

(a)  oesophagitis,
(b)  duodenitis,
(c)  gastritis,
(d)  posterior wall gastric ulcer,
(e)  anastomotic ulcer.

(3)  When on clinical grounds the irritable bowel syndrome is likely in a patient *under 30* it is important to make a positive diagnosis and in particular to exclude Crohn's disease.
The following investigations are suggested:

(a)  full blood count,
(b)  ESR,
(c)  barium follow-through,
(d)  sigmoidoscopy and rectal biopsy.

All should be normal in the irritable bowel syndrome.

(4)  In a patient *over 30* with symptoms suggestive of the irritable bowel syndrome, a double-contrast barium enema should precede the barium follow-through as it is important to exclude large bowel carcinoma in this age group.

(5)  If colorectal cancer is strongly suspected and has not been confirmed by sigmoidoscopy or barium enema, colonoscopy is indicated.

(6)  Gallbladder disease is confirmed by:
    (a)  an oral cholecystogram which will demonstrate stones or a non-functioning gallbladder,
    (b)  an ultrasound scan which, unlike the cholecystogram, will reveal stones even in the presence of jaundice.

(7)  Recurrent pancreatitis is often difficult to diagnose but most cases can now be confirmed by:

    (a)  measurement of the serum amylase during an attack of pain,
    (b)  ultrasound scanning,
    (c)  endoscopic retrograde pancreatography.

# 10

# Acute Diarrhoea

Acute diarrhoea can be subdivided into

(1) Acute infective diarrhoea
(2) Diarrhoea in travellers
(3) Diarrhoea due to drugs

## ACUTE INFECTIVE DIARRHOEA

The most frequent cause of acute diarrhoea is infection of the alimentary tract and is covered by the term 'gastroenteritis'. In these cases the associated symptoms of nausea, vomiting, lassitude, headache, fever and shivering all point to infection as the cause of diarrhoea. Although there is usually no problem in making the diagnosis of infective gastroenteritis, the aetiological agent is only rarely identified. The illness is almost invariably shortlived. Therefore, diarrhoea persisting without improvement for more than 2 weeks is unlikely to be due to infection. In these patients the causes discussed in Chapter 11, on chronic and recurrent diarrhoea, should be considered.

Numerous species of bacteria are known to be pathogens and more recently viruses have been implicated as an important cause of gastroenteritis, especially in children.

### Toxin-induced diarrhoea

*Staphylococcus aureus, Clostridia perfringens* and some strains of

83

*Escherichia coli* produce toxins which cause the small intestine to secrete large volumes of fluid. The colon is unable to compensate and watery diarrhoea results. Staphylococci and clostridia can cause diarrhoea without infecting the small intestine because their toxins are produced in contaminated food, prior to ingestion. In contrast *E. coli* have first to colonize the duodenum and jejunum before releasing toxins *in vivo*. Recent evidence suggests that the pathogenicity of *E. coli* depends upon the capacity of certain strains to adhere to the small bowel epithelium. This prevents the removal of the organisms by peristalsis and allows toxin to accumulate in high concentration close to the epithelium. Symptoms coming on within 2–6 hours of eating contaminated food are likely to be due to preformed toxin. Vomiting is frequently the first of these and may be the dominant feature. It is followed within a few hours by profuse diarrhoea and central abdominal colicky pain. The disease is short-lived and recovery is usually complete within 48 hours. Antibiotics are not indicated and in view of the brief nature of the condition, antidiarrhoeal preparations are rarely required. The patient can usually maintain adequate hydration and nutrition with glucose electrolyte solution, e.g. Dioralyte and Rehydrat. Very occasionally, toxin-induced diarrhoea may lead to sudden severe dehydration and circulatory collapse. This is particularly likely in the elderly, infants and those debilitated by other diseases. Such cases will need admission to hospital for intravenous therapy.

## Salmonella

The commonest species of Salmonella causing enteritis in man is *S.typhimurium*, but many others have now been identified. It must be remembered that the disease caused by these organisms varies greatly from those due to *S.typhi* and *S. paratyphi*. Typhoid and paratyphoid are characterized by bloodstream and widespread tissue invasion. Diarrhoea is not usually the main feature.

The exact mechanism whereby salmonella causes diarrhoea is not understood. However, in contrast to staphylococcal and clostridial toxin-induced disease, physical disruption and invasion of the intestinal epithelium occur. The ileum is the most severely affected but in some cases a colitis is also seen. Some strains of *E. coli* that do not produce enterotoxin may also cause diarrhoea by a similar mechanism. Infection usually results from contact with infected animals, meat, especially poultry which is insufficiently cooked (particularly deep-frozen varieties), and dairy products. Food may also be contaminated by human carriers. This type of infection is particularly common in communities, e.g. schools and hospitals. The incubation period is between 12 and 24 hours which helps to distinguish it from toxin-produced diseases. Symptoms include copious diarrhoea, often with blood and mucus, abdominal pain and vomiting. Accompanying fever and constitutional disturbance is common. Severe symptoms subside within 2–3 days but disturbed bowel habit may persist for 2–3 weeks. A fluid diet, antidiarrhoeal (codeine phosphate, loperamide and kaolin and morphine) and spasmolytic drugs (mebeverine and anticholinergics) help to keep the patient comfortable. Antibiotics are rarely indicated. In fact, the indiscriminate use of antibiotics in uncomplicated cases does nothing to shorten the course of the disease and may prolong the carrier state. Ampicillin or co-trimoxazole may, however, be needed for the rare case of severe infection which has led to prolonged constitutional disturbance and when bloodstream invasion has occurred. It is noticeable that achlorhydric patients suffer more severely, presumably owing to the lack of the protective action of hydrochloric acid.

## Shigella dysentery

*Shigella sonnei* and *flexneri* are by far the commonest causes of bacillary dysentery in the British Isles. The more severe disease caused by the *S.dysenteriae* species is usually contracted overseas. Infection spreads by contact with infected stool or articles that a patient has handled or worn, rather than from contaminated food or water. Outbreaks in schools or other institutions are common. The incubation period is 2–4 days. The main symptom is diarrhoea accompanied by blood and mucus. Lower abdominal pain, tenesmus, anorexia, vomiting and headache are also common. Examination reveals a mild-to-moderate pyrexia and diffuse abdominal tenderness without guarding. Because the large intestine is predominantly affected, an inflamed rectal mucosa on proctoscopy can be helpful in reaching a diagnosis. The disease is usually self-limiting and a glucose electrolyte solution and symptomatic treatment are all that are required. Antibiotics do not appear to reduce symptoms or eradicate the species of organism encountered in the British Isles and may propagate resistant strains. More severe forms contracted abroad need antibiotic treatment, preferably after tests on the patient's stools. The most useful antibiotics are co-trimoxazole, ampicillin, nalidixic acid and tetracycline. Admission to hospital is only necessary when dehydration threatens to lead to circulatory collapse and renal failure. Social conditions may also make domiciliary care impractical. However, when outbreaks occur in residential institutions it is probably wise to remove the initial victims. If the epidemic is uncurbed further evacuation is not indicated.

## Campylobacter

Only in the past ten years has the genus *Campylobacter* been implicated as a cause of enteritis. It is a vibrio-like organism. The exact mechanism by which diarrhoea is induced remains unclear, but it seems likely these organisms have the capacity to invade the gut mucosa. The small intestine is the principal site involved but a colitis may occur. Many animals harbour *Campylobacter*, including chickens, sheep, pigs, dogs and cats. Unpasteurized milk and untreated water have been implicated in some outbreaks. It is now the most commonly identified cause of adult infective enterocolitis in the British Isles. Unlike most enteric infections there is an incubation period of several days and diarrhoea is frequently preceded for 24–48 hours by prodromal symptoms. These are most commonly headache, myalgia, abdominal pains, pyrexia and shivering. Diarrhoea lasts for 2–3 days and is almost invariably accompanied by severe colicky abdominal pain. The stool is watery and sometimes contains blood. Lassitude and recurrent colic may persist for several weeks.

In a small number of cases the severity of abdominal pain and tenderness leads to an incorrect diagnosis of peritonitis and laparotomy. In others systemic disturbance, including arthritis, predominates. Fortunately most patients require only symptomatic management. The place of antibiotics is not clear but they should probably be reserved for the more severe cases. Erythromycin is the drug of choice.

Apart from shigellosis, bacterial diarrhoea is not usually transmitted from person to person. Because the pathogen is frequently contained in food many individuals may be affected simultaneously. When such outbreaks occur it is often possible to trace the origin of the contaminated food.

## Yersinia

*Yersinia enterocolitica* is now thought to play an important role in infective diarrhoea. It is found, like *Campylobacter* and *Salmonella*, in wild and domestic animals, unpasteurized milk, shellfish and water. Infestation often occurs as outbreaks in families and common sources of contaminated food have been found.

*Yersinia* is thought to act in a dual way. It produces an enterotoxin and also shows invasive properties particularly in the ileum, colon and mesenteric nodes.

Patients present with abdominal pain and diarrhoea with watery stools containing mucus. Blood is not common. About 50% of the patients are mildly febrile and the diarrhoea usually lasts for several days, but may continue occasionally for weeks. Due to the propensity for terminal ileitis the patients may undergo appendicectomy, when a thickened inflamed ileum, with enlarged mesenteric glands similar to Crohn's disease, is found. Occasionally the diarrhoea is accompanied by acute arthritis, thyroiditis, uveitis and erythema nodosum. Other manifestations are a generalized septicaemia and widespread abscesses.

Usually the enteritis is mild, probably undiagnosed and treated symptomatically. When the disease is systemic or there are severe bowel symptoms it should be treated actively. Tetracycline has been found to be useful for bowel symptoms and chloramphenicol is indicated for systemic disease.

## Virus infections

Virus infections of the gut tend to occur in epidemics. Schools and other similar institutions are particularly vulnerable, presumably because transmission of the organism is facilitated under these conditions. Many viruses have been implicated in epidemics of gastroenteritis but the two most consistently involved are rotaviruses and parvovirus-like organisms, which include the Norwalk agent. The former are almost certainly the commonest cause of childhood gastroenteritis in temperate climates.

As with the great majority of acute bacterial diarrhoeas, viral enteritis in adults is a shortlived disease and requires no more than domiciliary symptomatic management in most cases.

## DIARRHOEA IN TRAVELLERS

### Travellers' diarrhoea

All of the above bacterial causes of diarrhoea may be contracted in the British Isles but are more common in those countries where standards of hygiene and sanitation are poor.

It seems very likely that pathogenic *E. coli* are the commonest cause of diarrhoea in travellers to foreign countries, whether it be to Spain, Central America or the Middle East. The disease usually occurs within the first 2 weeks of arriving in the new country. Because it lasts for only 2–3 days most individuals have recovered by the time they return home. Prophylactic Streptotriad, one tablet twice daily, reduces the incidence of this disease. If the disease is more prolonged and persists after returning, shigella, or parasitic infestation should be considered.

### Giardia lamblia

By far the most likely parasite to cause diarrhoea in travellers is *Giardia lamblia.* It is endemic in the tropics, subtropical regions and the eastern Mediterranean. Outbreaks have also occurred in the USA and visitors to the USSR, particularly Leningrad, often return with this infestation. The organism is a flagellate protozoon which lives in human small intestine. Cysts are excreted in stool and infection occurs by ingesting contaminated food or water. Infestation is often asymptomatic; in those with symptoms there is a wide range of severity. Intermittent diarrhoea with abdominal discomfort and distention is common. In more severely affected cases the diarrhoea is profuse and significant malabsorption with weight loss can occur. Diagnosis is confirmed by the findings of cysts in the stool. Because these are not always present, examination of the duodenal fluid for trophozoites may be necessary to prove the diagnosis. Aspiration of duodenal fluid is usually combined with small bowel biopsy, sections from which will often reveal the organism between the villi. In severe cases there may be a mucosal abnormality with partial villous atrophy similar to that of tropical sprue.

Treatment is with metronidazole (Flagyl) 200 mg t.d.s. for 2 weeks or 400 mg t.d.s. for 1 week. The patients should be warned not to take alcohol with metronidazole because the drug has Antabuse-like effect.

## Amoebiasis

Infestation with *Entamoeba histolytica* is a rarer cause of diarrhoea in temperate climates than *Giardia lamblia*. Nevertheless, it is not exclusive to the tropics and is found in warm countries when sanitation and hygiene are poor. Infection occurs by ingestion of cysts which can contaminate water and food. The incubation period varies from a few weeks to several months. The disease may not manifest, therefore, until well after the patient has returned from his travels. In the majority of cases there is insidious onset of diarrhoea, the stool being mixed with blood and mucus. There is frequently no fever and only at a later stage does the patient complain of any systemic disturbance. Sigmoidoscopy shows scattered ulceration. Stool examination will reveal cysts and in fresh faeces it may be possible to see the motile trophozoites. Sections of a rectal biopsy should also be examined for trophozoites and the serum examined for antibodies to *E. histolytica*.

A small minority of patients have a more acute and severe disease. Their symptoms consist of bloody diarrhoea, fever and abdominal pain. Toxic dilatation of the colon is a rare complication in this group. Sigmoidoscopic appearances cannot be distinguished from idiopathic ulcerative proctocolitis. A history of travel and the relevant investigations are, therefore, vital in making a rapid diagnosis in such cases.

If untreated there may be spread of disease to cause an amoeboma or hepatic abscess. The most frequently used drugs are metronidazole and diloxanide furoate, which is particularly potent against cysts.

## Other parasites

Other parasitic infestations causing diarrhoea in patients returning to the British Isles are much less common. They include *Schistosoma mansoni*, tapeworms, *Ascaris lumbricoides*, hookworm, whipworm, *Trichinella spiralis* and *Strongyloides stercoralis*. In most cases examination of the stool will reveal the organism or its cysts. Sigmoidoscopy and rectal biopsy are particularly valuable in the diagnosis of schistosomiasis. When requesting stool examination for parasites it is important to state the countries in which the patient has stayed – even though the visit may have been many years in the past – because these parasites have characteristic geographical distributions.

## Tropical sprue

Tropical sprue must also be considered in those patients with diarrhoea returning from endemic areas. It occurs most frequently in south-east Asia and parts of the Caribbean. The characteristic features of tropical sprue are malabsorption in association with widespread partial villous atrophy of the small intestine. The aetiology is unknown but possibly results from combined nutritional deficiency and an altered microbial population of the gut. Clinical features are variable and apart from steatorrhoea and diarrhoea include megaloblastic anaemia, glossitis, pigmentation, abdominal discomfort and distension. Diagnosis depends on the appropriate history and jejunal biopsy. Many patients lose their symptoms on returning to a temperate climate. Others require long courses of treatment with folic acid and tetracycline.

## GUIDELINES FOR MANAGEMENT OF INFECTIOUS DIARRHOEA

Suggested guidelines are as follows:

(1)   Take stool, vomitus and suspected food to local microbiology laboratory.

(2)   Advise fluid diet and prescribe antidiarrhoeal and spasmolytic drugs when necessary.

(3)   Do not give antibiotics routinely.

(4)   Emphasize importance of strict hygiene to patient and relatives.

(5)   Admit to hospital if there is severe systemic disturbance, evidence of dehydration or other complicating disease.

(6)   In infants, seek paediatrician's advice in all but the mildest cases.

(7)   In cases where the organism has been identified, or where a common source of infection seems likely, notify the local health authority.

(8)   Instruct anyone who handles food that they may not do so until their stools are free of the pathogen.

## DIARRHOEA DUE TO DRUGS

Acute diarrhoea may be caused by drugs of many different categories. It is, therefore, very important to review current and recent drug regimes in any patient presenting with diarrhoea.

### Antibiotic-induced diarrhoea

Other than laxatives, antibiotics are the therapeutic agents that most often cause this problem. Most patients have only mild bowel disturbance and the disorder usually passes within 2–3 days of stopping the antibiotic.

### *Pseudomembranous colitis*

The most serious form of antibiotic-induced diarrhoea is pseudomembranous colitis. This disorder, as its name implies, is an inflammatory disease of the large intestine. Sigmoidoscopy reveals the characteristic pseudomembrane overlying an oedematous hyperaemic mucosa. Histology shows areas of intense but superficial ulceration. The pseudomembrane consists of epithelial debris, fibrin and leukocytes. In the most severe cases microthrombi and crypt abscesses are seen. The lesion is often patchy; a single biopsy, therefore, may not be representative. The diarrhoea consists of profuse liquid stool which sometimes contains blood. Other features, which include colic, pyrexia and leukocytosis, vary greatly in severity. In some cases intensive intravenous therapy is needed to correct dehydration, electrolyte imbalance and hypoproteinaemia. On rare occasions a toxic megacolon develops which may necessitate colectomy. The symptoms can commence within the first few days of antibiotic treatment, but onset is more usual between the fourth and tenth days. It is, nevertheless, important to realize that symptoms may not start until 3 weeks after antimicrobial drugs have ceased. This latter group frequently have a more severe and protracted illness.

Many patients who develop pseudomembranous colitis have other debilitating diseases or have recently undergone surgery. It seems likely that a serious illness itself can be responsible for pseudomembranous colitis because there have been a few documented cases in which antibiotics have not been involved.

The antibiotics most often implicated are clindomycin, lincomycin and ampicillin, but there have been sporadic reports which throw suspicion on many others.

The cause of this disease in the great majority of cases is a toxin produced by *Clostridium difficile*. It seems probable that antibiotic therapy either renders the colonic mucosa more vulnerable to the toxin or enhances the proliferation of *C. difficile* by reducing the numbers of other organisms. In many patients whose diarrhoea starts whilst on antibiotics, stopping the drug results in cure. In those whose symptoms start or persist after stopping the offending antibiotic, vancomycin 150 mg four times daily, or metronidazol 400 mg t.d.s. should be given.

In the past *Staphylococcus aureus* was considered to be the cause of pseudomembranous enterocolitis. Proven staphylococcal enterocolitis is now very rare and it seems likely that many cases previously attributed to this organism were really due to *C. difficile*. It is not known if the very common, mild and rapidly resolving attacks of antibiotic-induced diarrhoea are also due to *C. difficile* toxin or whether other mechanisms are involved.

## Other drugs causing diarrhoea

There can be few drugs that have not been blamed for causing diarrhoea. In the situation where symptoms have coincided with starting a new drug it is wise, where possible, to stop it and change to an alternative preparation. Drugs that often cause diarrhoea include carbenoxylone and other liquorice derivatives, antacids containing magnesium salts, digoxin (at toxic levels) mephanamic acid (Ponstan), indomethazine (Indocid), guanethidine (Ismelin), methyldopa (Aldomet) colchicine and the majority of cytotoxic agents. In addition to causing diarrhoea some drugs may also cause malabsorption. Amongst these are neomycin, cholestyramine, phenindione and para-aminosalicylic acid.

# 11

# Chronic Diarrhoea

The term 'diarrhoea' is best restricted to describing the passage of large amounts of poorly formed stool. Most viral and bacterial diarrhoeas rarely last for more than a few days and *if diarrhoea continues for more than 2 weeks infective diarrhoea is unlikely*. *Giardia lamblia* and *Entamoeba histolytica* are exceptions to this (see Chapter 10).

For the purposes of this discussion, 'chronic' is defined as longer than 2 weeks. Many patients will have a much longer history and may well have suffered recurrent attacks over several years.

The common causes of chronic diarrhoea are:

(1)   the irritable bowel syndrome,

(2)   chronic inflammatory bowel disease,

(3)   carcinoma of the large intestine,

(4)   malabsorption.

More than 90% will be due to one of these disorders.

## TIMING OF DEFAECATION AND DESCRIPTION OF STOOL

The passing of a 'normal' stool followed by several poorly formed stools *soon after waking* is characteristic of the irritable bowel syndrome. Absence of symptoms at weekends and when on holiday is common in this condition, suggesting that stress is a major factor in many patients. *Urgency of defaeca-*

*tion within minutes of a meal* is also typical of the syndrome but in many there is no fixed pattern. Some patients with inflammatory bowel disease have an increased frequency of defaecation in the mornings, but most have bowel disturbance throughout the day. *Nocturnal defaecation* is rare in the irritable bowel syndrome and when this is present inflammatory bowel disease must be seriously considered.

*Large amounts of stool*, particularly when liquid (more than 400 mg or ml per day) is most likely to be due to inflammatory bowel disease or malabsorption. Many patients with the irritable bowel syndrome do not have true diarrhoea but merely *frequency of defaecation*. In such cases the stool is characteristically pellety or ribbon shaped weighing only a few grams. The sensation of *incomplete rectal emptying* is also common in this group but is also present in proctitis, rectal cancer and faecal impaction.

Stool containing *blood and mucus* is an indication of organic disease such as proctocolitis, neoplasia or diverticular disease. *Bloodstaining of the toilet paper only* is most likely to be due to piles or a fissure, but this must not be assumed without full examination of the rectum both digitally and endoscopically.

*Mucus, but not blood, coating the stool* is frequently found in the irritable bowel syndrome but when there are large amounts colorectal tumours or inflammation must be sought for.

*Steatorrhoea* will usually present as diarrhoea and only rarely will the patient give the 'textbook' description of a pale, bulky, offensive and floating stool. *Most stools that float contain an excess of gas and not of fat and do not indicate steatorrhoea*. 'Silver' stool is due to bloodstaining of the steatorrhoea and is usually due to cancer of the head of pancreas.

Whenever possible the stool should be examined. This frequently necessitates *admission to hospital* when it is usually possible to rapidly distinguish patients with true diarrhoea from those who have merely frequency of defaecation.

## ALTERNATING DIARRHOEA AND CONSTIPATION

A history, extending over several years, of erratic bowel habit with episodes of frequency of defaecation followed by constipation is typical of the irritable bowel syndrome. By contrast a similar pattern involving only a few weeks or months may be due to carcinoma of the large bowel.

Many elderly patients who are severely constipated have episodic and often profuse *spurious diarrhoea*. Incontinence is commonly due to seepage of liquid stool around faeces impacted in the rectum or sigmoid colon. The problem is made worse by the taking of stimulant laxatives and can only be

94

solved by clearing the rectum. This can sometimes be achieved with stool softeners (dioctyl sodium sulphosuccinate) and washouts. In many cases only manual removal is successful. *Carcinoma of the rectum or left side of the colon and sigmoid diverticular disease may also cause spurious diarrhoea.*

## ADDITIONAL SYMPTOMS

Although diarrhoea may be the dominant symptom, attention should be paid to other clinical features.

*Weight loss* without anorexia may indicate small bowel disease, chronic pancreatitis or thyrotoxicosis.

*Anorexia* accompanying diarrhoea in the over-40 age group raises the suspicion of large bowel carcinoma. Crohn's disease and lymphoma are more likely causes in younger age groups.

*Abdominal pain and discomfort*, usually in the lower abdomen, are symptoms of the irritable bowel syndrome. There are often two distinct components; one is a persistent generalized ache or sensation of distension; the second is a more sporadic severe colic often associated with defaecation. Confusingly, patients with Crohn's disease and bowel cancer may experience similar symptoms. *Travel*, particularly when recent, may be important and stools should be searched for *Giardia lamblia* and *Entamoeba* cysts.

*Drugs and alcohol* are common causes of diarrhoea. Enquiry should be made about proprietary medicines including laxatives and herbal preparations based on senna or liquorice and antidyspepsia mixtures containing magnesium salts. Non-steroidal anti-inflammatory drugs, especially mefanamic acid (Ponstan), may be responsible for profuse diarrhoea. Unfortunately, some patients who take laxative preparations will not admit to doing so (*see below*, on surreptitious laxative abusers). Abuse of alcohol disturbs bowel function, but patients often refuse to attribute the diarrhoea to their drinking habits.

## PHYSICAL EXAMINATION

*Thorough examination of all patients with chronic diarrhoea is mandatory.* A routine examination that reveals no abnormality does not, of course, eliminate organic disease and if the history has already raised definite suspicions it will still be necessary to investigate.

*An abdominal mass* in a patient with diarrhoea is likely to be due to colonic carcinoma, Crohn's disease or small bowel lymphoma.

*Tenderness and definite guarding* may be present in Crohn's disease and diverticulitis. It seems unlikely that uncomplicated diverticulosis causes diarrhoea. However, incomplete sigmoid colon obstruction with spurious diarrhoea due to luminal narrowing is a well recognized complication of the disorder.

Tenderness without true guarding is common in the irritable bowel syndrome when it is often possible to palpate a 'spastic' sigmoid colon.

*Pyrexia* is usually an indication of inflammatory disease and is most often due to Crohn's disease or diverticulitis.

*Digital examination of the rectum* is obligatory. Blood on the glove confirms the need for more extensive investigation, because of the possibility of either neoplastic or inflammatory bowel disease. In many cases the site of bleeding will be piles or diverticular disease. Either of these conditions, when accompanying the irritable bowel syndrome, can therefore be confused with more sinister pathologies such as carcinoma and inflammatory bowel disease. The majority of rectal carcinomas can be felt within the lumen and many cancers of the sigmoid will also be palpable extrinsic to the rectal wall. Perianal fissures, fistulae and fleshy skin tags favour the diagnosis of Crohn's disease.

*Anaemia* is not a feature of the irritable bowel syndrome and when it is present cancer, inflammatory disease and malabsorption must be excluded. Other signs of malnutrition such as *glossitis*, *angular stomatitis*, *oedema* and *musculoskeletal pain* may also occur in the malabsorption syndrome.

*Lymphadenopathy* in the supraclavicular fossae might indicate metastatic spread of large bowel carcinoma, whereas more generalized enlargement of lymph nodes may be an indication of lymphoma.

---

- Frequency of defaecation restricted to the period soon after rising is usually due to the irritable bowel syndrome

- Diarrhoea with weight loss, blood per rectum or anaemia requires early investigation

- Rectal examination will diagnose a high proportion of colorectal cancers and lead to early surgical referral

---

## INVESTIGATION

*Sigmoidoscopy* must be performed in chronic diarrhoea. *Endoscopy of the rectum can be carried out easily in the surgery or outpatient clinic without need of bowel preparation.* Only very young children, the rare extremely anxious patient and those with painful anal fissures require sedation or anaesthesia. Sigmoidoscopy and biopsy will confirm the diagnosis of rectal carcinoma.

Examination of the mucosa *combined with biopsy* will provide a definite diagnosis in virtually all cases of ulcerative proctocolitis and in many with Crohn's disease. In ulcerative colitis the rectum is uniformly involved. The lesion ranges from hyperaemia and oedema to granularity in the mild and moderately affected cases. In severe disease there is spontaneous bleeding and disruption of the mucosa. When the condition is restricted to the rectum (proctitis) it may be possible to get above the involved segment and view normal mucosa. Crohn's disease frequently spares the rectum. In other cases of Crohn's disease there are patches of inflammation and discrete ulceration. Aphthous-type ulcers of the rectal mucosa are also found in this condition. A cobblestone appearance of the mucosa is another characteristic feature of Crohn's disease. Amoebic colitis cannot be distinguished readily from these two conditions on naked eye appearances. Thus, those who have been to areas where this disease is endemic must also have the appropriate stool and serological tests. Even when no definite lesion can ben seen, blood or excessive mucus coming from above the endoscope indicates that there is need for continuing investigation.

*Culture and examination of the stool* for bacterial pathogens and parasites should be arranged. However, with the exception of *Mycobacterium tuberculosis* and possibly *Shigella*, bacteria do not cause chronic diarrhoea. By contrast, infestation with *Entamoeba histolytica* commonly goes on to cause chronic bowel disturbance. The former should be suspected in patients from developing countries who complain of bloodstained diarrhoeal stool. It is essential that fresh faeces are examined when looking for pathogenic amoeba. A serological test is now also available and is positive in a high percentage of cases.

Another protozoan, *Giardia lamblia*, may also cause chronic diarrhoea and sometimes steatorrhoea. It infests the small intestine and it is, therefore, best confirmed by examination of duodenal juice obtained by intubation. This procedure is often combined with small bowel biopsy. Stool examination for the *G. lamblia* ova is also positive in a smaller proportion of patients.

*Occult bleeding* should be sought for when there is no clear evidence of rectal blood loss. Providing piles and anal fissure have been excluded, a positive test is likely to be due to inflammatory disease, neoplasia or diverticular disease.

*Simple blood tests* will often make discrimination possible between patients with the irritable bowel syndrome and those with more serious intestinal disease. A normal haemoglobin concentration and white cell count, together with an erythrocyte sedimentation rate in single figures, though not excluding organic disease, favours the diagnosis of the irritable bowel syndrome. A low haemoglobin in patients with diarrhoea may be the result of intestinal neoplasia, ulcerative colitis, Crohn's disease or small bowel malabsorption.

In patients with chronic diarrhoea a low serum albumin level is most likely to be due to excessive gut loss of protein. Active widespread inflammatory bowel disease is the commonest cause. It may also result from coeliac disease and small bowel lymphoma. In rare instances large amounts of protein can be lost from a large bowel carcinoma. Normal plasma protein levels are found in the irritable bowel syndrome.

When small bowel malabsorption is suspected, a low red cell folate and serum vitamin $B_{12}$ level would encourage definitive investigation which would include a barium follow-through examination and small bowel biopsy.

If these simple investigations prove unfruitful, before arranging radiological studies it is worthwhile considering the following causes of diarrhoea:

thyrotoxicosis,
diabetes mellitus,
carcinoid syndrome,
surreptitious laxative abuse.

*Thyrotoxicosis* causes diarrhoea by increasing small bowel motility and reducing the gut transit time. It is easily confirmed by simple thyroid function tests.

*Diabetes mellitus* is occasionally complicated by diarrhoea which is often nocturnal. The mechanism is not entirely clear, but is probably partly due to an autonomic neuropathy of the gut leading to abnormal motility. There may be an alteration in gut bacterial flora and disturbance of bile salt metabolism. Treatment is frequently ineffective. Some patients respond to simple antidiarrhoeal agents and others benefit from courses of broad spectrum antibiotics. Recently cholestyramine, a substance which binds bile salts and interferes with their cathartic action on the intestine, has proved useful.

*Carcinoid syndrome* is a very rare cause of profuse diarrhoea. Carcinoid tumours of the small intestine, when they metastasize to the liver, procude large quantities of 5-hyrox tryptamine, kallikrein and prostaglandins. These substances affect gut function and lead to diarrhoea which may be continuous or episodic. The accompanying features of flushing, dilation of skin blood vessels, asthma and signs of pulmonary and tricuspid valvular disease of the heart support the diagnosis. Elevated levels of 5-hydroxyindolacetic acid in the urine are confirmatory. Treatment includes symptomatic relief with 5-hydroxytryptamine antagonists. In some cases it is possible to enucleate the secondary tumours from the liver. Cytotoxic drugs infused into the hepatic artery and therapeutic embolization of this vessel may also give symptomatic relief. The tumour is slow growing and 50% of patients can be expected to live for 5 years or longer from the time of presentation.

*Surreptitious laxative abusers* often present with diarrhoea. Even when confronted with a daunting programme of investigation the majority do not volunteer that purgatives are being used. Other symptoms include abdominal discomfort and distension, thirst, lethargy, muscle weakness, due to dehydration and hypokalaemia. Less commonly, steatorrhoea and protein-losing enteropathy occur and clubbing, osteomalacia and oedema may also be present.

The patient is usually female and invariably psychologically disturbed. Many have coexistent anorexia nervosa, and the abuse of other drugs, especially diuretics, is common. Denial of purgative usage hinders diagnosis and it is usually necessary to arrange hospital investigation to exclude other causes of metabolic disturbance. Such patients go to extraordinary lengths to conceal their actions. In hospital it may be necessary to search their lockers for purgatives and to test the stool for phenolphthalein and the urine for anthraquinone metabolites. Management is extremely difficult and depends mainly upon treatment of the underlying psychological disorder. Some authorities believe there is little to be gained by a confrontation with the patient. This frequently results in her moving from one doctor to another or the precipitation of some other form of psychological disturbance.

## Radiology

This will be necessary in the majority of patients with chronic diarrhoea. When clinical and investigatory evidence points to chronic pancreatic disease calcification may be seen within the gland on straight abdominal X-ray. If small bowel malabsorption is suspected small bowel biopsy should be requested before barium studies, as the majority of such cases in Europe and North America will have coeliac disease which can only be diagnosed conclusively by histology.

Chronic diarrhoea with bleeding per rectum must be investigated by double-contrast barium enema. Many patients will have no more than the irritable bowel syndrome with coincidental piles, diverticular disease or a colonic polyp, but it is imperative to exclude carcinoma and inflammatory disease. Even when endoscopy has demonstrated carcinoma or inflammatory disease of the rectum, barium enema is essential to exclude synchronous tumours or to define the extent and distribution of the inflammatory lesion.

In patients with anaemia or a raised erythrocyte sedimentation rate, a barium enema is also indicated. If this examination is negative and Crohn's disease is suspected, a barium follow-through should be arranged.

If there is no evidence of intestinal bleeding and the rectal biopsy, stool and blood tests are normal, the decision whether to arrange barium studies is more difficult. In patients over the age of 30 it is wise to proceed to a barium enema in order to exclude carcinoma. In those under 30 the barium enema is not so immediately vital, because cancer of the large intestine is extremely unlikely. It must be admitted that this plan of investigation will undoubtedly delay the diagnosis in a small number of patients with Crohn's disease. Nevertheless, it is extremely unlikely that these cases will be in jeopardy providing they are kept under review and investigated further if symptoms worsen or new signs develop.

## Colonoscopy

This is indicated in patients when investigation points to either large bowel carcinoma or inflammatory disease, but double contrast barium enema and sigmoidoscopy have failed to confirm the diagnosis. This procedure has now become widely available. The new fibreoptic instruments permit a thorough examination of the entire large bowel and tissue can be obtained for histology. The colon must be clear of faeces; this can be achieved by a number of different techniques. Most centres use a liquid diet for 48 h before examination combined with purgation or colonic lavage. Parenteral sedation and analgesia are given immediately prior to the examination. As with upper gastrointestinal endoscopy the patient is able to return home later the same day.

# 12

# Malabsorption

There are numerous mechanisms that cause the malabsorption syndrome.

*Intrinsic widespread disease of the small intestinal mucosa* as found in coeliac disease and tropical sprue causes malabsorption due to reduced digestive and absorptive function of the epithelial cells.

*Resection of the small intestine* because of trauma, inflammation, neoplasia or vascular disease decreases the total area available for absorption. Long segments of small bowel may be removed with little effect upon nutrition because there is a large reserve capacity. Furthermore the remaining small bowel hypertrophies and increases its ability to absorb.

Vitamin $B_{12}$ and bile salts are specifically absorbed from the terminal ileum. Disease or resection of this part of the intestine, most commonly due to Crohn's disease, often gives rise to a macrocytic, megaloblastic anaemia. Bile salt malabsorption is the other serious consequence. These substances are produced in the liver and pass via the biliary system into the duodenum. They act as detergents and allow the products of fat digestion to mix with water in the gut lumen. This involves the formation of aggregates called mixed micelles. This process facilitates the absorption of fatty acids, monoglycerides and fat soluble vitamins from the duodenum and jejunum. The bile salts themselves are not absorbed at these sites but are released from the micelles into the lumen. This enables them to be reutilized, if necessary, throughout the length of the small intestine. They are eventually actively absorbed from the terminal ileum and pass via the circulation to the liver, from where secretion into the biliary system again takes place. This conservation is essential because the liver has a very limited capacity to synthesize bile salts. When bile salt absorption is impaired, due to disease or resection of the ileum, recirculation is interrupted. This causes bile salt deficiency with a reduction in micelle formation and malabsorption of fat and fat soluble vitamins. In this situation bile salts pass into the colon where they have a potent cathartic action. Such patients, therefore, suffer from both steatorrhoea and diarrhoea.

*Gastric surgery* is a common cause of minor degrees of malabsorption. The mechanisms (Figure 12.1) include:

inadequate mixing of food with digestive juices in the stomach,
rapid gastric emptying,
release of pancreatic enzymes and bile, uncoordinated with gastric emptying.
bacterial colonization of the upper small bowel after a Polya gastrectomy.

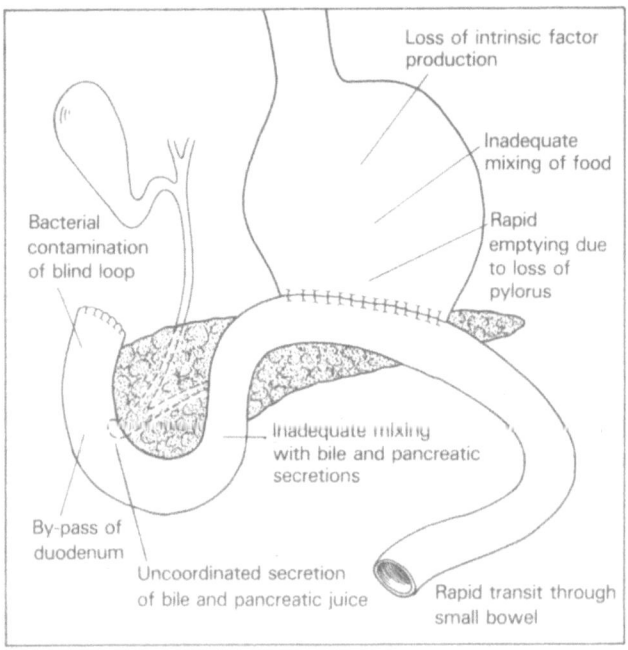

**Figure 12.1** Mechanisms of malabsorption after gastric surgery (from Lancaster-Smith, M. (1983) *Peptic Ulcer*. (London: Update Publications))

*Colonization of the small intestine by bacteria.* Any condition that allows small bowel stagnation or contamination encourages excessive proliferation of bacteria. These include:

diverticulosis,
enterocolic fistulae,
scleroderma,
amyloidosis.

Faecal bacteria, especially Bacteroides, degrade bile salts causing depletion of these vital compounds and *E. coli* interfere with the absorption of vitamin $B_{12}$.

*Pancreatic insufficiency*, usually due to chronic pancreatitis, causes malabsorption because there is a deficiency of enzymes to digest the large molecular constituents of food prior to absorption.

*Hepatic and biliary disease* may result in inadequate quantities of bile salts reaching the small intestine. It is very rare for hepatic or biliary disease to cause significant malabsorption in the absence of jaundice. Thus, this cause of malabsorption is easily identified and does not pose a diagnostic problem.

The common causes of malabsorption in the United Kingdom are:

gastric surgery (p. 54)
coeliac disease (p. 108)
Crohn's disease (p. 122)
chronic pancreatitis (p. 109)

Much rarer causes are intestinal resection, lymphoma, chronic intestinal ischaemia, radiotherapy damage, infestation with Giardia, tropical sprue and Whipple's disease.

## CLINICAL FEATURES

Malabsorption usually presents with one or more clinical features which individually are often unimpressive. When they occur in combination, malabsorption should be suspected.

### Diarrhoea and steatorrhoea

Inspection of the faeces is of great importance. However, the pale, floating bulky, offensive steatorrhoea stool said to be typical of malabsorption is rare. *Furthermore the absence of even mild diarrhoea does not exclude malabsorption*. Frank or occult blood loss may be found in Crohn's disease or lymphoma.

## Abdominal pain

Generalized abdominal discomfort and distention is common. Chronic pancreatitis causes persistent bouts of dull upper abdominal pain often interspersed with short attacks of more severe pain which radiate to the back. Colic may indicate intermittent obstruction of the small intestine due to Crohn's disease or, more rarely, lymphoma. An inflammatory or neoplastic mass may be palpable in such patients.

## Nutritional deficiency

Severe nutritional deficiency is extremely rare. In contrast, mild deficiency of several nutrients is common and should always raise the possibility of malabsorption.

*Weight loss* is due partly to inadequate absorption but in some conditions such as Crohn's disease and lymphoma increased catabolism and anorexia contribute.

*Anaemia* is by far the commonest presenting nutritional deficiency. It may present indirectly with tiredness, dyspnoea or angina but often it comes to light during routine blood tests. In severe cases angular stomatitis and glossitis occur. In coeliac disease and postgastrectomy patients *iron deficiency* is common. Bleeding may contribute to iron deficiency following gastrectomy, due to reulceration, and in those with Crohn's disease and lymphoma.

*Macrocytic anaemia* is caused by *folate or vitamin $B_{12}$* deficiency. Because folate is mainly absorbed in the upper small intestine, low levels are very common when the jejunum is the major site of pathology, as in coeliac disease. In Crohn's disease low folate levels are due to a combination of malabsorption, inadequate intake and increased metabolic utilization caused by the inflammatory nature of the disorder. Vitamin $B_{12}$ is absorbed by the terminal ileum and, thus, longstanding disease or resection of this part of the intestine will inevitably give rise to deficiency. It is particularly common in Crohn's disease. Vitamin $B_{12}$ malabsorption may also occur when there is stasis in the small intestine. This results because the proliferating bacteria metabolize the vitamin within the lumen of the bowel before it can be absorbed. The commonest causes of stasis and bacterial contamination of the small intestine are Polya gastrectomy, strictures and fistulae, usually due to Crohn's disease, and small bowel diverticulosis. A combined lack of iron and folate or vitamin $B_{12}$ leads to a dimorphic blood film. This should always raise the suspicion of malabsorption and stimulate a search for its cause.

104

*Bone pain due to osteomalacia and weakness of proximal limb muscles* as a result of *myopathy*, both caused by malabsorption of vitamin D, are found in small numbers of patients. Serum calcium levels are frequently normal or only marginally lowered, but the alkaline phosphatase is often raised. A minority have significantly reduced serum levels of calcium and present with *tetany*.

A slightly increased prothrombin time due to malabsorption of vitamin K may occur, but only very rarely is the deficiency severe enough to cause pathological *bruising*.

*Low serum albumin levels* in malabsorption can occasionally be severe enough to cause *oedema*. This is partly caused by malabsorption of peptides and amino acids but is frequently due to loss of protein from the diseased intestine. This is termed *'protein-losing enteropathy'* and is most commonly found in coeliac disease, Crohn's disease or lymphoma. It is not exclusive to small bowel disease and sometimes occurs with carcinomas of the stomach and colon or ulcerative colitis.

*Peripheral neuropathy* and *mental dysfunction* have been reported especially in coeliac disease but the mechanism is obscure. Similarly, other symptoms of malabsorption such as *lethargy and lack of energy* cannot be attributed to any particular nutritional disturbance. They are likely to be the result of multiple minor deficiencies and electrolyte depletion.

## Other signs

*Clubbing* of the finger nails and *skin pigmentation*, in conjunction with the above features, though relatively rare, should increase the suspicion of small bowel disease. Patients with an irritant vesicular rash should be suspected of having *dermatitis herpetiformis* which is usually accompanied by the small bowel lesion of coeliac disease.

*Additional features* from the past or present history may be invaluable in preventing unnecessary investigation in patients suspected of malabsorption. These include:

previous gastric surgery or intestinal resection,

abdominal or pelvic irradiation,

prolonged diarrhoeal illness in childhood suggesting coeliac disease,

foreign travel raising the possibility of tropical sprue or giardiasis,

alcohol abuse causing damage to small intestine or chronic pancreatitis,

diabetes mellitus,

scleroderma which causes malabsorption due to small bowel stagnation.

## Investigation

It is usual to support the suspected diagnosis with a few simple non-invasive investigations. These include:

a full blood count, which may show signs of iron, folate or vitamin $B_{12}$ deficiency,

low levels of serum folate or red cell folate,

a reduced serum albumin concentration,

low levels of serum calcium and elevation of alkaline phosphatase.

*It must be emphasized that some patients with malabsorption will not be distinguished by these simple tests.*

## Small bowel biopsy

Because coeliac disease is the commonest cause of clinically significant malabsorption in the British Isles a small bowel biopsy is now normally performed at this stage. This avoids multiple unnecessary tests in the great majority of patients with malabsorption. Numerous capsules and tubes are available for obtaining small bowel biopsies but the most frequently used is the Crosby capsule or one of its modifications. The capsule and attached tube are swallowed and manoeuvred under radiological screening into the proximal jejunum. Alternatively the capsule may be passed in conjunction with a fibreoptic endoscope. The latter method enables rapid positioning of the capsule and the entire procedure rarely takes more than 10 minutes. It is well tolerated and the incidence of complications is very low.

In coeliac disease the biopsy will characteristically reveal subtotal villous atrophy.

Other *much rarer* conditions that can be regularly diagnosed by small intestinal biopsy include:

tropical sprue,
amyloidosis,
intestinal lymphangiectasia,
Whipple's disease,
*Giardia lamblia* (examination of intestinal fluid for trophozoites is also important).

Crohn's disease and lymphoma may also occasionally be confirmed by this technique.

## Xylose absorption test

If small bowel biopsy facilities are not readily available, or when the suspicion on clinical and haematological grounds is not so great, the *xylose absorption test* can provide helpful information. Xylose is a pentose which is readily absorbed from the small intestine. It is not metabolized in the body and is excreted unchanged in the urine. Both blood levels and the amount excreted in the urine after oral ingestion are measured. Used in this way the test will detect the great majority of patients with coeliac disease. This is because the diffuse lesion of the small intestine causes impaired absorption with resulting low blood and urine levels. By contrast, xylose absorption is usually normal in Crohn's disease in which the lesion is patchy or restricted to the terminal ileum. Similarly, in malabsorption due to pancreatic disease because the small intestine is normal, xylose absorption is unimpaired.

## Antireticulin antibody

Another test that is useful in adding weight to the suspicion of coeliac disease is the antireticulin antibody test. It employs immunofluorescence to detect antibodies in the serum of patients with coeliac disease and is present in approximately 75% of untreated cases. *However, it must be emphasized that no other test can substitute for the small bowel biopsy in the diagnosis of coeliac disease.*

## Radiology

If the small bowel biopsy does not achieve a diagnosis, a barium follow-through examination is justified to look for evidence of anatomical abnormality.

The conditions most likely to be confirmed by the examination are:

Crohn's disease (strictures and fistulae; p. 124)
small bowel diverticulosis
lymphoma
gastric and bowel resections

## Faecal fat

When the above investigations have failed to provide a diagnosis, but malabsorption is still suspected, faecal fat estimation is indicated. A 5-day collection is necessary as there is wide daily variation of fat excretion. The test is delayed in the hope that it will not be required because it usually necessitates admission to hospital and collection of stools is unpopular with patients, nurses and laboratory staff. Nevertheless, the demonstration that a patient exretes an average of more than 6 g of fat per day, whilst taking between 70–100 g of fat in the diet, is good evidence of malabsorption and will encourage a continuing search for its cause.

## COELIAC DISEASE

Coeliac disease is by far the commonest cause of clinically significant malabsorption in developed countries. In the United Kingdom about one in two thousand of the population develop the disease. There is an increased family incidence but the exact mode of inheritance is not known.

The disease is caused by the gliadin fraction of gluten which in some way is 'toxic' to the small bowel. Existing evidence suggests that there is an abnormal immunological reaction in response to gliadin leading to the characteristic villous atrophy of the small intestinal mucosa.

*Diagnosis can only be made by small bowel biopsy* and noting the clinical, biochemical and histological response to treatment with a gluten-free diet.

A gluten-free diet involves avoidance of products made with wheat, barley and rye flour. Most patients tolerate oats and maize is certainly safe. A large variety of gluten-free foods are now on the market many of which are obtainable in the UK on NHS prescriptions.

Most patients who adhere to their diet do not need maintenance nutritional supplements, although iron and folate may be necessary initially to replenish depleted stores.

A few adult patients fail to respond to a gluten-free diet alone but do so when small doses of prednisolone are given.

Coeliac disease in adult life is associated with an increased incidence of:

- small intestinal lymphoma and carcinoma
- oesophageal carcinoma
- pancreatic insufficiency
- splenic atrophy
- small bowel ulceration
- auto-immune diseases

Strict adherence to a gluten-free regime does not seem to affect the incidence of these complications.

## Dermatitis herpertiformis

This skin condition is characterized by an irritant vesicular rash and in the majority of sufferers there is a gut lesion comparable to that of coeliac disease. Although bowel symptoms and nutritional disturbance are uncommon, a gluten-free diet is now often advised because both the rash and villous atrophy are responsive to this treatment. The alternative therapy for the rash is Dapsone but this has no effect on the bowel abnormality.

## MALABSORPTION DUE TO PANCREATIC DISEASE

If there is steatorrhoea but:

(1)  no history of gastric or bowel resection
(2)  no previous irradiation of pelvis or abdomen
(3)  a normal small bowel biopsy
(4)  a normal barium follow-through

the likely diagnosis is *chronic pancreatitis*. The following tests are used to support the diagnosis of chronic pancreatitis:

(1)  serum amylase – which may be raised during acute exacerbations

(2)  glucose tolerance test – which is diabetic in 60%

(3)  abdominal X-ray – shows calcification of the gland in 30%

(4)  pancreatic function tests

   (a)  measurement of bicarbonate and enzymes in duodenal aspirate following secretin and pancreozymin infusion
   (b)  measurement of enzyme concentration in duodenal aspirate after stimulation of pancreas with a standard Lundh meal

(5)  endoscopic retrograde pancreatography will show dilated, tortuous or strictured ducts – calculi or cysts may also be visualized

(6)  ultrasound scanning and computerized axial tomography may show abnormal morphology

## BACTERIAL CONTAMINATION OF SMALL INTESTINE

When the history or radiological studies suggest bacterial proliferation as a possible cause of malabsorption, the following tests are often employed to support the diagnosis:

(1)  the radioactive carbon bile salt breath test, which depends upon excessive bacterial deconjugation of labelled bile salt, the radiocarbon from

109

which is excreted as carbon dioxide in the breath, where it can be measured

(2) urinary indican estimation gives a semiquantitative estimate of the intestinal metabolism of tryptophan, which is increased in small bowel bacterial contamination

### Vitamin $B_{12}$ malabsorption

Intrinsic factor is produced in the gastric mucosa and is essential for the specialized absorption of vitamin $B_{12}$ from the terminal ileum. In pernicious anaemia, atrophy of the gastric glands leads to deficiency of intrinsic factor which, in turn, causes malabsorption of vitamin $B_{12}$. Malabsorption of vitamin $B_{12}$ also occurs when the terminal ileum is diseased or has been resected. A third mechanism for the malabsorption of vitamin $B_{12}$ is seen in small bowel stagnation. Under these circumstances the excess bacteria, usually *E. coli*, metabolize the vitamin before it can be absorbed from the terminal ileum.

*The Schilling test* is a means of measuring vitamin $B_{12}$ absorption. A small amount of radioactively labelled vitamin $B_{12}$ is taken orally, followed by a large intramuscular dose of non-labelled $B_{12}$. This cause vitamin $B_{12}$, including the labelled portion, to be flushed from the body. The amont of labelled $B_{12}$ excreted in the urine over the next 24 hours is proportional to the amount absorbed. If the test has been performed correctly and kidney function is normal, a low urinary excretion of radioactive label indicates malabsorption of vitamin $B_{12}$. In pernicious anaemia this can be corrected by the addition of exogenous intrinsic factor (part 2 Schilling test). This does not, of course, correct malabsorption of vitamin $B_{12}$ when it is caused by disease or resection of the ileum or small bowel bacterial overgrowth. If bacterial overgrowth is the primary reason for malabsorption of vitamin $B_{12}$ it is frequently improved after a course of broad spectrum antibiotic therapy (part 3 Schilling test).

---

- Diarrhoea and steatorrhoea are not always present in the malabsorption syndrome

- Anaemia is the commonest presenting feature of small bowel malabsorption

---

# 13

# The Irritable Bowel Syndrome

In the past the irritable bowel syndrome has been called by a variety of names including mucous colitis, spastic colon, colonic dysfunction and the splenic and hepatic flexure syndromes.

The exact prevalence is unknown but a recent survey suggests that up to 15% of the population intermittently suffer from symptoms compatible with the diagnosis. It is by far the commonest cause of referral to gastroenterologists. Twice as many females as males have the condition which mostly presents in the third and fourth decades.

## AETIOLOGY AND PATHOGENESIS

Many studies have shown moderate degrees of anxiety and depression in those presenting with the disorder. Approximately 50% will have identified stress as an important precipitating factor of their attacks, but in many sufferers psychogenic mechanisms seem to be less important.

Eating may precipitate symptoms but it is rarely possible for patient or doctor to implicate specific dietary items. There is much current debate about the role of food 'allergy' in the irritable bowel syndrome but as yet the evidence is far from convincing. Nevertheless a small number of patients in whom diarrhoea is the main symptom benefit from avoiding milk because they have coexistent alactasia. This occurs because undigested lactose on entering the colon has a cathartic action. Lack of dietary fibre has been implicated as an important factor and may well be so when constipation is the principal feature.

Gastrointestinal infections and infestations are commonly followed by prolonged bouts of disturbed bowel function, which fulfill the diagnostic criteria of the irritable bowel syndrome.

The autonomic nervous system, local neurotransmitters and hormones all have an effect upon colonic muscle activity. Motility of the colon during an exacerbation of the irritable bowel syndrome is abnormal. Those whose main symptoms are pain and constipation have an excess of non-propulsive segmenting contractions. In those with diarrhoea there is a decrease in this type of activity. It seems likely that pain comes from distension of the bowel proximal to the area of increased segmentation. Distension of the colon and even small intestine by balloons precipitates pain in patients with the irritable bowel syndrome more readily than in non-sufferers. This suggests that there may be a reduced threshold to pain perception in this condition. Patients who experience pain after meals have an abnormal colonic response to cholecystokinin which is released into the blood when food enters the duodenum. It seems that the fundamental abnormality in the irritable bowel syndrome may be a difference in the basal electrical activity of the smooth muscle when compared to normal. This, apparently, makes the colonic muscle more susceptible to nervous and humoral stimuli, which could explain why stress and meals are common exacerbating factors. Studies on the oesophagus and small intestine in patients with the irritable bowel syndrome show abnormal motility in these organs, indicating that there may be a widespread abnormality of smooth muscle function in this condition.

## CLINICAL FEATURES

There are three main clinical categories.

### Pain with erratic bowel habit

This is by far the largest group. Pain is most frequently felt in the lower abdomen and is usually described as a constant ache often interspersed with bouts of more severe colic. Partial relief is afforded by passing stool or flatus, but in some patients this may precipitate pain. Bouts of constipation are common, whilst at other times frequency of defaecation is the main problem. True diarrhoea rarely occurs and the stool is usually described as pellets, bits and pieces or ribbon shaped. Coating with mucus is not uncommon.

### Postprandial pain

Another category includes those in whom pain is frequently precipitated by meals. Because of this there may be confusion with peptic disease. In contrast to gastric or duodenal ulcer, however, the pain is rarely confined to the epigastrium and the characteristic one-finger localization of the site by the patient is not elicited. Furthermore, the symptom is more usually described vaguely as a discomfort rather than true pain. Again in contrast to duodenal ulcer, nocturnal pain is rare. When pain is experienced in the right or left hypochondria the terms 'hepatic' and 'splenic' flexure syndromes are often used.

### Painless diarrhoea

In about 10% of patients with the irritable bowel syndrome, diarrhoea without pain is the predominant symptom. This problem is frequently at its worst soon after rising in the morning and after breakfast. In many an initial normal stool is followed by numerous poorly formed motions.

Other symptoms that commonly accompany the pain and bowel dysfunction of the irritable bowel syndrome include:

the sensation of abdominal distension,
what the patient believes is excessive flatulence,
nausea without vomiting

Examination is usually unremarkable, but in some patients it is possible to palpate a 'spastic' pipe-like left colon. Rectal and sigmoidoscopic examination are normal.

The full blood count, erythrocyte sedimentation rate, rectal biopsy and barium enema show no abnormality.

## MANAGEMENT

The most important aspect of management is to make a positive diagnosis on the clinical evidence.

It is also essential to perform the few relevant investigations listed above. This has two main purposes – to exclude more serious gastrointestinal disease and to add power to your reassurance. The patient should be given an adequate explanation of the disorder (*see Appendix 1* Information for Patients) and must *not* be told 'there is nothing wrong' or given the impression that he or she is imagining the symptoms. It is worthwhile making specific mention that the condition has no connection with colitis or cancer and that it does not progress to more serious bowel disease.

### Psychological factors

Recognition that stress is a factor can sometimes help, as may the intermittent use of mild tranquillizers, such as diazepam (Valium) and lorezepam (Ativan). Accompanying depression frequently responds to tricyclic drugs. Because of their anticholinergic activity they may also have a direct beneficial effect upon colonic smooth muscle dysfunction.

## Diets

When specific foods precipitate symptoms they should clearly be avoided. However, most patients with the disorder are unable to identify a close or consistent relationship to dietary items. It is, therefore, rarely justifiable to subject them to complicated exclusion diets.

When constipation is the predominant feature, an increase in dietary fibre should be tried. Bran-containing cereals and wholemeal bread are acceptable means of achieving this. Some patients find bran and bran-containing products unpalatable or inconvenient and in this circumstance one of the proprietary products, such as Fybogel, Normocol or Regulan, is a suitable alternative. Unfortunately, increased dietary fibre frequently exacerbates pain and the sensation of distension. This often decreases if the patient perseveres, but many are unable or unwilling to do so. When constipation is not a significant feature increasing dietary fibre will rarely be helpful. By contrast, if colicky pain and distension are the predominant problems a low residue diet during severe attacks will often provide rapid relief from symptoms.

## Antispasmodic drugs

Oral anticholinergic drugs are usually disappointing. This is almost certainly because the dosage necessary to relax colonic muscle causes unacceptable side-effects such as dry mouth, blurred vision, bladder dysfunction and drowsiness. Nevertheless, during severe bouts of pain many patients are willing to endure these in order to obtain relief. The drugs most commonly used are propantheline (Probanthine), hyoscine (Buscopan), dicyclomine (Merbentyl) and slow release atropine (Peptard). Merbeverine (Colofac) has a direct antispasmodic action on colonic smooth muscle and has no significant anticholinergic effects. It is therefore usually more acceptable, and seems to be particularly useful taken before meals in those who suffer from postprandial pain. The dosage is 135–270 mg.

## Antidiarrhoeal drugs

If soft, poorly-formed stools are the major symptom, codeine phosphate, diphenoxylate (Lomotil) and loperamide (Imodium) will usually help.

Because diarrhoea is often at its worst on rising, a regular dose at night is often beneficial.

## Conclusion

*Patients with the irritable bowel syndrome must be warned that it is a chronic remitting and relapsing condition for which, as yet, there is no cure.* Many will continually return to their own practitioner for reassurance, whilst others over the ensuing years will seek further numerous opinions. Repeated unnecessary investigation should be resisted.

# 14
# Ulcerative Proctocolitis and Crohn's Disease

There is now a body of opinion which holds that ulcerative proctocolitis and Crohn's disease represent variants of a single disorder which can reasonably be termed *'idiopathic inflammatory bowel disease'*. In this chapter, however, the two diseases are discussed separately, although it is admitted that there are a considerable number of cases in which despite clinical, radiological and pathological information, it is impossible to achieve a categorical diagnosis.

## ULCERATIVE PROCTOCOLITIS

Ulcerative colitis occurs most frequently in white races but is becoming more common in the developing countries of Asia and Africa. All age groups are affected. The prevalence in Britain is approximately one per 1200 of the population. There is an undoubted increased incidence in some families but it is not known whether the predisposition is genetic or environmental.

### Aetiology and pathology

The cause of ulcerative colitis is not known. It seems very likely that the disease may be due to an abnormal immunological response either to a bacterium or virus, which has yet to be identified. The condition might then become a self-perpetuating auto-immune disorder because the immune system fails to suppress the inflammation. In the past psychosomatic mechanisms have been implicated but there is no good evidence to support this.

117

The rectum is almost invariably diseased and is usually most severely affected. The inflammation may be confined to the rectum – the condition is then correctly described as *non-specific or idiopathic proctitis*. In other cases the disease may affect only the rectum and left colon, whilst many even at presentation have total large bowel involvement. *The small intestine is always spared*.

Severity of inflammation varies widely, ranging from diffuse erythema to frank ulceration and pseudopolyps. In longstanding cases the colonic mucosa becomes pale and featureless. Fibrosis causes shortening and narrowing but, unlike Crohn's disease, strictures are rare. The histological features include a cellular infiltrate of plasma cells, neutrophils and eosinophils, crypt abscesses in the mucosal glands and depletion of goblet cells. In contrast to the inflammatory reaction of Crohn's disease, the muscle and serosal layers are not involved. Diarrhoea results, owing to a combination of transudation of fluid across the inflamed mucosa and a failure to absorb water and electrolytes by the damaged colon.

## Clinical features

*Diarrhoea* is the predominant symptom. Its onset may be sudden and violent but is more commonly insidious and recurrent. Several episodes may occur before presentation or diagnosis is made. *Blood and mucus* intimately mixed with the stool are characteristic. When the disease is restricted to the rectum tenesmus, urgency of defaecation and bleeding are the usual symptoms and true diarrhoea does not occur. *Abdominal discomfort* related to bowel action is common but severe pain is very unusual. Fulminant cases have fever, dehydration and severe constitutional disturbance.

In patients with only proctitis, there are no abnormal physical signs other than the typical sigmoidoscopic appearance of the rectum. In contrast, severe cases are frequently anaemic, dehydrated and pyrexial. *Abdominal tenderness and distension indicate severe disease*. The latter is due to dilatation of the colon which may perforate.

## Diagnosis

Diagnosis of proctocolitis can be confirmed in general practice by proctoscopy. A normal rectal mucosa for all practical purposes excludes proctocolitis. *Sigmoidoscopy* allows a more extensive examination of the rectum and biopsy of the mucosa will provide unequivocal evidence of inflammatory disease. The extent of disease must be assessed either by barium enema or colonoscopy.

## Management

### Proctitis

Proctitis is brought under control with local steroid preparations such as prednisolone suppositories or enemas (Predsol, Predenema, Colifoam). Sulphasalazine (Salazopyrin) 1 g twice daily should be started at the same time and continued for a minimum of 12 months to reduce the risk of relapse.

Although outpatient attendance will usually be necessary to establish the diagnosis, these patients do not require longterm follow-up at hospital, providing their disease remains confined to the rectum. However, it should be remembered that 10% will eventually develop colitis, and for this group long term hospital follow-up is essential.

### Colitis

Colitis is defined as inflammation extending above the rectum.

### Mild to moderate disease

This is characterized by

passage of fewer than six stools per day,
no systemic symptoms and
no excessive blood loss,

and is not an indication for immediate admission. But an urgent appointment for *medical* outpatients must be arranged. After confirmation that the patient has inflammatory disease, oral prednisolone 15 mg twice daily and sulphasalazine 2–3 g daily should be started without delay.

Effectiveness of treatment is judged by a reduction in stool frequency and the sigmoidoscopic appearance of the rectum. Once remission has been achieved the dose of prednisolone should be gradually reduced and stopped after a period of 6–8 weeks. The incidence of relapse is unaffected by long term low dose prophylactic steroid therapy. *In contrast sulphasalazine 1 g twice or three times daily unequivocally reduces the chance of relapse* and should probably be continued indefinitely. A small number of patients are unable to take sulphasalazine because of unwanted effects. Most are due to hypersensitivity to the sulpha radical. The commonest is skin rash and only rarely are more serious problems, such as thrombocytopaenia and anaemias encountered. The drug may cause gastric irritation but this can usually be overcome by prescribing enteric coated tablets and reducing the dose, and by the patient taking it with meals.

119

A new preparation, 5-aminosalicylic acid, which does not contain the sulpha radical, will soon be available to general practitioners, and trials have shown that it is at least as effective as sulphasalizine in preventing relapse.

Codeine phosphate and loperamide give useful symptomatic relief during the first few days of a mild or moderate relapse until steroid therapy has induced remission. Long term use is sometimes necessary when complete remission is not achieved.

## Severe disease

Patients who in their first or subsequent attacks have

systemic disturbance,
severe bleeding,
more than six stools per day,

are classified as having severe disease and should be admitted to hospital.

Inpatient care should be directed by a physician but close consultation with a surgeon experienced in colonic surgery should be maintained throughout the initial period of treatment. These patients will have variable pyrexia, electrolyte and fluid depletion and anaemia. Treatment includes correction of the metabolic disturbance and anaemia with blood and appropriate intravenous fluids. Steroids should be administered parenterally (prednisolone 80 mg intravenously per day, or adrenocorticotropic hormone (ACTH) intramuscularly 80 units daily or tetracosactrin acetate (Synacthen) intramuscularly 1 mg daily). Nutrition can be maintained intravenously or by enteral tube feeding. The great majority of patients treated by this regimen show a significant improvement within 5 – 7 days. They can then be allowed a low residue diet and parenteral steroids are replaced with oral prednisolone 40 – 60 mg daily. This is gradually reduced and sulphasalazine is given, as previously described, for longterm prophylaxis.

Those patients who, on the above regimen, show no improvement within the 5 days, or actually deteriorate and particularly if they develop toxic dilatation, are treated by urgent colectomy. Assessment during this period includes close monitoring of temperature, pulse rate, 'well-being' and the amount and frequency of stools. The abdomen should be examined at least twice daily for evidence of dilation or perforation. *It must be kept in mind that steroids may disguise the symptoms and signs of perforation and peritonitis.*

## Long term management

All patients with ulcerative colitis, as distinct from proctitis, should be kept under regular review in a hospital outpatient department, preferably by a physician with a major gastroenterology interest. Only a small minority have a single attack. More commonly the course is one of remission and relapse.

Despite continuous sulphasalazine and courses of steroids a few patients will have uncontrollable symptoms and colectomy must then seriously be considered. Another factor that favours surgical intervention is recurrent active disease for more than 10 years, because this confers a 30 times greater chance of developing large bowel cancer than that of the general population (Figure 14.1).

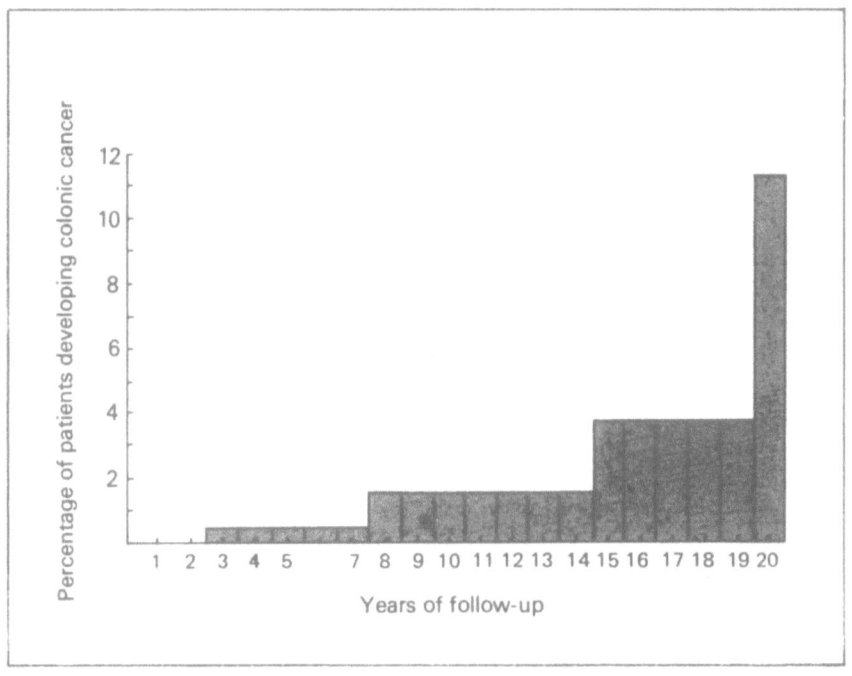

**Figure 14.1** Cumulative risk in ulcerative colitis of developing colonic cancer (Radcliffe Infirmary, Oxford) (from Lancaster-Smith, M. and Williams, K. (1982) *Problems in Gastroenterology*. (Lancaster: MTP Press))

In addition to clinical assessment, the haemoglobin, liver function and plasma protein levels should be checked at least annually. It is now also common practice to examine all longstanding cases every 12 – 24 months by colonoscopy. This may detect early carcinoma but additionally multiple biopsies are obtained which may show premalignant dysplasia. If dysplastic changes are found in a patient whose disease is disrupting his life, the decision to proceed to colectomy is not difficult. By contrast, when dysplasia coexists with inactive disease the decision is more contentious, as such patients are naturally reluctant to undergo colectomy.

Patients with longstanding disease are now commonly followed-up in a 'colitis clinic' run jointly by a physician and surgeon. This makes possible the development of rapport and undoubtedly facilitates making major decisions such as the need for colectomy. Proctocolectomy is the usual operation in such cases, although many surgeons do this in two stages. The first consists of colectomy and fashioning an ileostomy. At a later stage the rectum is removed. In a minority the rectum subsequently heals sufficiently for it to be anastomosed to the ileum (ileorectal anastomosis), thus dispensing with the ileostomy. A few surgeons advocate colectomy and ileorectal anastomosis as a primary procedure. Recurrent active disease and the potential risk of cancer in the rectum are the main reasons why this operation is not more popular.

## CROHN'S DISEASE

As with ulcerative colitis, Crohn's disease most commonly occurs in white races. All age groups are affected, but the onset is seen most frequently in early adult life. However, there appears to be an increasing incidence in adolescence. By contrast to ulcerative colitis, Crohn's disease has become more common during the past 20 years, and in the United Kingdom is found in 1 in 4000 of the population. There is an increased family incidence but it is not clear whether this is entirely due to genetic factors.

### Aetiology and pathology

The cause of Crohn's disease is unknown. Current evidence suggests that it may be due to a micro-organism. This is largely based on experiments which have shown that homogenates of bowel affected by Crohn's disease cause Crohn's-like lesions when injected into animal tissues. Furthermore, the lesion can be passaged from one animal to another. It is not known whether the putative organism is a virus or bacterium. *Acute ileitis* is commonly caused by infection with *Yersinia enterocolitica* or *Yersinia pseudotuberculosis*. However, as only a tiny number of patients with acute ileitis go on to develop chronic disease it is very unlikely that Yersinia is the cause of Crohn's disease. There have been many attempts to demonstrate that patients with Crohn's disease have an impaired immunological status, but results are conflicting. Nevertheless, present knowledge suggests that patients with Crohn's disease may have a disturbed immune response to antigens of varying origin that have penetrated the gut mucosa.

There is recently published evidence that smoking may protect against developing ulcerative colitis and that the contraceptive pill may increase the chance of contracting Crohn's disease. Those who believe that the two conditions are different forms of a single disorder have subsequently hypothesized that these environmental factors may merely modify the immune response in inflammatory bowel disease and determine whether the patient develops 'ulcerative colitis' or 'Crohn's disease'.

Unlike ulcerative colitis, the disease may involve any part of the alimentary tract from mouth to anus. The terminal ileum and caecum are most commonly affected. Lesions of the small and large intestine are often multiple and separated by mucosa of normal appearance. Although a continuous disease in the colon is not uncommon, the rectum is frequently spared, which again contrasts with the characteristic distribution in ulcerative colitis. Ulceration of the mucosa varies from superficial aphthoid lesions to deep ulcers that penetrate the submucosal layers. Adjacent loops of bowel become adherent and fistulae are common. Fibrosis is often dense which leads to stricture formation. Histology shows transmural inflammation and fissures. In more than 50% of cases non-caseating granulomas can be found.

## Clinical features

The predominant symptoms of Crohn's disease are abdominal pain, diarrhoea and general malaise. Pain may vary from vague discomfort, often after food, to severe colic due to a degree of intestinal obstruction. Diarrhoea occurs in a smaller proportion of patients than in ulcerative colitis but may be accompanied by steatorrhoea if there is significant small bowel involvement. Identifiable blood is seen in the stool when the large bowel is predominantly affected. Weight loss and other features of malabsorption, particularly anaemia, are common.

Perianal ulcers, fissures, fistulae, abscesses and fleshy skin tags surrounded by bluish-brown skin are characteristic. An abdominal mass, especially in the right iliac fossa, or signs of small bowel obstruction may occur. Nevertheless, it must be stressed that early in the course of the disease there are frequently no definite clinical features and because of this definitive diagnosis is often delayed for many years.

## Diagnosis

As with ulcerative colitis, *sigmoidoscopy* is mandatory. Endoscopic appearances vary from patchy erythema and discrete ulceration to diffuse inflammation but, because the rectum is often spared, a normal appearance does not exclude Crohn's disease. However, biopsies obtained even when the mucosa appears macroscopically normal may show typical submucosal inflammation.

*Barium follow-through* may reveal mucosal ulceration and strictures. The *barium enema* in Crohn's colitis shows deep fissures and a cobblestoned appearance of the mucosa. It is also the best method of demonstrating fistulae between large and small intestine.

*Colonoscopy* is now widely available and is an even more accurate means of assessing the severity and distribution of the inflammation in the large intestine and terminal ileum.

## Management

### Acute attacks

The initial attack and subsequent relapses require treatment with steroids. The regimen is similar to that used in ulcerative colitis. The effect is often less dramatic in Crohn's disease and more prolonged courses are frequently needed.

*Pain* is often an indication of reactivity and will then usually respond to steroid therapy. However, pain may occur even when Crohn's disease is inactive, from partial obstruction of the intestine due to fibrosis. The erythrocyte sedimentation rate or C reactive protein estimation are helpful in such cases. Pentazocine and Temgesic are useful drugs. They are conventionally combined with antispasmodics, but efficacy of these drugs is unproven.

*Anaemia, electrolyte,* and *nutritional disturbances* must be treated by transfusion and appropriate supplements. In patients with extensive small bowel involvement or resection, those with enteral fistulae, or when steroids fail to induce a remission, tube feeding or parenteral feeding may be necessary.

Intra-abdominal and perineal *abscesses* are treated with appropriate antibiotics such as a combination of co-trimoxazole 2 tablets b.d. and metronidazole 400 mg t.d.s.

## Prophylaxis

*Prevention of exacerbations is the major problem in the management of Crohn's disease. Salazopyrin* is often used in large bowel Crohn's disease but it is certainly less effective than in ulcerative colitis. In a recent trial, *azathioprine (Imuran)* was shown to reduce the relapse rate significantly, and it deserves further assessment. Scandinavian studies suggest that metronidazole also has a place in preventing relapse.

## Surgery

*Because surgery is eventually necessary in approximately 75% of patients with Crohn's disease, combined long term management by a physician and surgeon is advisable.*

The reasons for surgery are:

(1)   the relief of acute intestinal obstruction,

(2)   drainage of an abscess,

(3)   resection of gut involved in fistulae between other segments of gut, bladder, vagina and skin,

(4)   resection of a stricture that is causing recurrent bolus colic or a stagnant loop,

(5)   haemorrhage or perforation,

(6)   colitis unresponsive to medical treatment, especially when toxic dilation is threatening.

Resection of affected gut is the usual procedure and bypassing of diseased bowel is no longer favoured.

## Long term management

Crohn's disease is a chronic relapsing condition. Nevertheless, most patients are able to lead a relatively normal life. All patients with inflammatory bowel disease should be instructed to seek medical advice at the first suggestion of a relapse because prompt action at this stage will often prevent a serious exacerbation. Most gastrointestinal units offer an urgent appointment on demand. The shortcomings of management are exemplified by the facts that patients treated medically have symptoms in 4 out of every 5 years, and following surgical resection there is a 50% chance of relapse within 10 years and in many a further operation will be necessary.

*Nutritional status* should be assessed at least annually. Iron, folate and vitamin $B_{12}$ deficiency are particularly likely in those with small bowel disease or resection. Diarrhoea does not necessarily indicate reactivation of the disease and may be due to a stagnant loop or bile salt catharsis. Whatever the mechanism small regular doses of codeine phosphate or loperamide are extremely useful and safe even for long term usage. A low fat diet is worthy of trial as is cholestyramine 4 g b.d. when bile salts catharsis due to ileal resection or small bowel stagnation is suspected.

Both small and large bowel *cancer* are increased in Crohn's disease compared to the general population. However, the risk of developing colonic carcinoma does not appear to be as great as in ulcerative colitis.

## EXTRA-INTESTINAL COMPLICATIONS

Apart from the bowel complications, both ulcerative colitis and Crohn's disease are associated with extra-intestinal problems. The frequency of these is thought to be lower in Crohn's than ulcerative colitis. The following are the most common.

### Arthritis

Transient non-erosive arthritis occurs in approximately 10%, sacroileitis in 20% and ankylosing spondylitis in 5%. The activity of the arthritis usually runs parallel with that of the bowel disease and responds to steroid treatment.

### Skin disease

A history of cutaneous vasculitis which most commonly takes the form of erythema nodosum is found in 10%, whereas pyoderma gangrenosum is much rarer. Vasculitis responds to steroid therapy but pyoderma gangrenosum is often unresponsive. In a few cases colectomy alone is successful.

### Ophthalmic disease

Conjunctivitis and uveitis often accompany arthritis and occur in about 5%. They are usually responsive to steroids.

The exact aetiology of the joint, cutaneous and ophthalmic complications is unknown, but they are likely to be due to circulating immune complexes that have been stimulated by gut luminal antigens crossing the diseased mucosa.

126

## Liver disease

A wide range of liver disorders is found in inflammatory bowel disease. The association is stronger in ulcerative colitis but even in this condition chronic hepatic disease giving rise to symptoms is rare. Of these pericholangitis is the commonest, but primary sclerosing cholangitis, chronic active hepatitis, biliary carcinoma and cirrhosis are also found. The pathogenesis of these hepatic disorders is not clear. Immune complexes again may be involved. Alternatively, bacteria or their toxins could readily cross the damaged bowel and via the portal vein pass to the liver. Colectomy, therefore, is often advised in cases of progressive liver disease.

## Gallstones and renal stones

In chronic Crohn's ileitis there is an increased incidence of gallstones. This occurs because the enterohepatic circulation of bile salts is interrupted. As a consequence certain bile salts are depleted, which leads to cholesterol crystallization in the gallbladder. Oxalate absorption is increased in inflammatory disease of the ileum, which predisposes to the formation of renal calculi. The mechanism of the increased absorption is unknown.

## SPECIAL PROBLEMS

### Disease in childhood

Diagnosis is frequently delayed in children, usually because the possibility of ulcerative colitis or Crohn's disease is not considered. Both the medical and the surgical management of acute inflammatory bowel disease in children are the same as that outlined for adults. In Crohn's disease, because courses of steroids are often more prolonged, there is a danger of stunting growth. This can be minimized by giving the steroid on alternate days or as a single morning dose.

### Pregnancy

Crohn's disease or ulcerative colitis do not adversely affect established pregnancy. Because sulphasalazine has no apparent teratogenic effect it may be continued. Steroids should be used for acute exacerbations. First attacks of colitis starting in pregnancy are notoriously severe. There is no increased rate of relapse during pregnancy in either condition but the puerperium is often associated with an exacerbation.

# 15

# Diverticular Disease of the Colon

Diverticula are small outpouchings of colonic mucosa. In Western society they are found in approximately 40% of those over 60 years of age.

## AETIOLOGY AND PATHOGENESIS

Why diverticula form is unknown but, because of the association with increasing age, degenerative processes are probably involved. Disordered colonic motility with excessive segmented contractions have been found in several studies. Because the disease is rare in the developing world and common in Europe and North America, a refined low roughage diet has been implicated.

## CLINICAL FEATURES

Presentation before the age of 50 is very uncommon. Only about 25% of those with diverticula in the colon experience symptoms that can be attributed definitely to the lesions. Patients undergoing investigation for the irritable bowel syndrome are often found to have diverticula but it is most unlikely that they are in any way responsible for symptoms such as vague abdominal discomfort, flatulence and erratic bowel habit.

Diverticular disease can usefully be divided into *diffuse* and *sigmoid* diverticulosis. In *diffuse diverticulosis* the lesions are found throughout the colon and tend to be shallow with wide mouths. By contrast *sigmoid diverticulosis* is confined to that part of the colon. The diverticula are long with narrow necks.

## Colic and large bowel obstruction

A characteristic of sigmoid diverticular disease is progressive hypertrophy of the colonic smooth muscle which leads to marked narrowing of the lumen. This causes colicky pain, often accompanied by severe constipation. This may occasionally be sufficiently severe to cause large bowel obstruction.

## Bleeding

Blood that is readily identified by the patient is a common presenting symptom of either diffuse or sigmoid diverticular disease. In the former bleeding is often massive. Blood may be passed alone or mixed with stool.

## Perforation

Perforation in diffuse diverticulosis usually leads to generalized peritonitis with the characteristic features of severe pain, guarding and systemic disturbance. Perforation of a sigmoid diverticulum is more likely to be confined and result in a pericolic abscess (*see below*).

## Diverticulitis

Stasis in a diverticulum predisposes to *inflammation*. The term diverticulitis should be reserved for this condition. Pyrexia, malaise and lower abdominal pain are the major symptoms. Examination reveals definite tenderness and guarding. An inflamed diverticulum may *perforate* causing a localized pericolic abscess when, on rectal examination, it is often possible to palpate a tender extrinsic mass. Generalized *faecal peritonitis* following perforation is relatively rare. Spread of infection to the bladder gives rise to *frequency of micturition* and *dysuria*. This may progress to a vesicocolic *fistula* giving rise to pneumaturia. Fistulae may also develop between the colon and vagina causing *vaginal discharge*. A fistulous tract between large and small intestine, although relatively rare, may cause a *stagnant loop syndrome* and *malabsorption*.

## Management

Colonic diverticula are confirmed and alternative disorders are excluded by barium enema. The examination will also permit assessment of the extent and severity of the disease. It has been claimed that increasing dietary fibre will decrease diverticula formation, but there is no evidence that this is so. However, when *constipation* is the predominant symptom increasing dietary fibre may be helpful, as may the occasional use of other laxatives.

Pain due to spasticity of sigmoid colonic muscle can be eased by adequate doses of mebeverine or anticholinergic drugs combined with suitable analgesia (pentazocine, aspirin or paracetamol). Opiate derivatives, such as morphine and codeine, should be avoided as they enhance colonic contractions and increase intraluminal pressure. Pain is also often dramatically eased by adopting a low residue diet for a few days.

*Acute diverticulitis* must be treated with a broad spectrum antibiotic such as amoxicillin (Amoxil) or co-trimoxazole (Septrin). A strict fluid diet should be adopted and antispasmodics and analgesics given as described above. Many patients can be treated at home on this regimen but if there is no improvement within 48 hours admission is advisable.

Other absolute indications for admission are:

massive bleeding
intestinal obstruction
perforation
abscess
fistula

Surgery will usually be necessary in such cases. Primary excision of the diseased segment may be possible. This is usually combined with a temporary colostomy, reanastomosis being left to a second operation. In many patients excision is not possible and all that can be offered is peritoneal toilet and a transverse colostomy. The diseased segment is subsequently resected when the inflammation has settled and the patient's condition has improved. Resection will also be necessary if a fistula has formed and in those experiencing recurrent severe inflammatory exacerbations.

The place of *elective surgery* in diverticular disease is not clear. Some surgeons will resect a severely hypertrophied section of the sigmoid colon when this is causing bouts of severe colic or obstruction. An alternative to resection is *sigmoid myotomy*. In this operation the circular colonic muscle is divided longitudinally. Although this lowers intraluminal pressures symptoms often return 2–3 years later.

Patients with diverticular disease should be given a simple explanation of their condition (see Appendix information sheet) and strongly reassured that they do not have cancer.

# 16

# Constipation and other Problems with Defaecation

## CONSTIPATION

It is important to realize there is wide variation in the frequency of defaecation. Nevertheless, 90% of the population in the United Kingdom open their bowels between five times per week and twice per day. Only 1% has two or fewer bowel actions per week. Many of this latter group do not, however, have symptoms referable to constipation and doubtless accept their habit as normal. In contrast, there are many who quite naturally have a more frequent bowel action yet consider themselves constipated because they do not have a daily movement. This misconception often stems from childhood and the rigid attitude of parents to toilet training. Constipation is, therefore, difficult to define but is probably best used to describe the *infrequent production of hard stool which requires excessive straining to pass*.

The great majority of patients presenting with constipation have no associated disease. This is termed *'simple' constipation*. Many have excessive segmenting movements of the colon which restrict the passage of stool and others appear to have reduced peristaltic movements. The mechanisms that control this smooth muscle activity are not understood. It seems likely that future research may reveal abnormalities of electrical activity and local neurotransmission. Whatever the mechanism, there is little doubt that lack of dietary fibre, inactivity and old age exacerbate the problem. Many patients with constipation have repeatedly *ignored the urge to defaecate* when the rectum is filled from the colon by peristalsis. This, in due course, leads to reduced sensitivity of the defaecating reflex. Increasing distension of the rectum is required to elicit the urge sensation which is eventually lost.

133

In such cases rectal examination frequently reveals a loaded rectum. In the majority of patients who deny this urge the reasons are sociological rather than medical. These include embarrassment in requesting to leave class-rooms and places of work and dislike of public lavatories. Other patients may have a painful local condition of the anus, such as fissure or piles and, therefore, try to pass stool as infrequently as possible.

There is an increased incidence of constipation in *pregnancy* but it is not clear whether this has a hormonal or mechanical basis. In a small minority of patients, constipation may be a presenting or complicating feature of other disorders. Constipation is often a prominent symptom of the *irritable bowel syndrome*. The diagnosis is suggested by alternating diarrhoea and constipation, variable abdominal pain, the absence of blood loss per rectum and insignificant constitutional disturbance (Chapter 3).

## The management of simple constipation

Attention to those factors known to exacerbate constipation are often all that is needed. Patients should, therefore, be advised to increase the intake of fibre by including wholemeal bread, All-Bran or bran itself in their diet. Taking additional fluid and exercise will also help. It is most important that the patient is instructed to respond appropriately to the defaecation urge. He or she should also be reassured that a daily bowel action may not be normal for them and that there is no need to resort to potent laxatives if this is not achieved.

## Special problems

### Faecal impaction

Impaction of stool in the rectum or even sigmoid colon is the result of severe constipation. The main complaint may be of diarrhoea or incontinence due to seepage of fluid stool around the impacted mass. The problem is particularly likely to arise in the elderly, bedridden patients and paraplegics. A stool softening agent, such as the dioctyl preparations, or olive oil as an enema should be used initially. These may be followed by stimulant laxatives such as Dulcolax and Senokot by mouth or glycerine or Dulcolax by suppository. If rectal loading persists, digital removal will be necessary. When the colon as well as the rectum is loaded, sodium phosphate enemas are of value.

### Maintenance regimes

Simple constipation will usually require no more treatment than previously discussed. Some patients will, nevertheless, require supplementary dietary fibre in order to maintain satisfactory bowel action. There are numerous preparations available of which Fybogel, Normacol, Metamucil and Isogel are the most commonly used. Despite all of these measures one is left with a small number of patients who require some additional help. It is not clear whether they are a specific subgroup who have an, as yet, undefined disturbance of colonic function. An osmotic purgative, such as lactulose, should be tried first but if this fails it may be necessary to allow the occasional use of stimulant laxatives such as Senokot and Dulcolax.

## Prophylaxis

Those undergoing surgery or other treatment for piles or fissure will need to keep their stools soft and thus avoid unnecessary pain. As this is a short term problem the choice of agent is not critical.

It is wise to anticipate that enforced immobility, especially in the elderly, is likely to precipitate constipation. Preparations such as Milpar and lactulose are useful for this purpose.

## Inappropriate use of laxatives

Many patients become convinced that they have an 'unsatisfactory' bowel habit and as a consequence resort to using laxatives on a regular basis. By the time she, or more rarely he, presents, there is a long history of taking laxatives, to which the patient will freely admit. They will complain that without laxatives no stool is passed for many days or weeks. Some resort to purgatives under these circumstances because with increasing constipation they experience abdominal pain and distension. Others wrongly attribute a multitude of symptoms, such as headaches and lethargy, to their sluggish bowel function. Some patients, however, have no accompanying symptoms but take laxatives as a habit because they firmly believe that a daily bowel movement is essential to health. This belief and ritual laxative usage has often started in childhood or adolescence. The majority have become dependent upon the chemical stimulant purgatives which include the anthraquinones (senna, cascara and danthron) or polyphenols (phenolphthalein and bisacodyl). Long term use of these drugs damages the myenteric plexus of the colon which is probably the reason that increasing doses are required with chronic usage. The history of constipation, interspersed with bouts of passing poorly formed stool, should always raise the possibility of large bowel cancer, even when the patient admits to recurrent use of laxatives. This is especially so in those over 40 years of age. Sigmoidoscopy and barium enema should, therefore, be performed. In purgative users radiology will often reveal a featureless colon and in some there will be the characteristic smooth pseudostrictures of a cathartic colon. Sigmoidoscopy may show melanosis coli which appears like dark freckles. They are due to lipofuscin contained in mucosal macrophages.

There are two main aims of management.

(1) The first is to convince the patient that daily defaecation is not essential and that there is a wide variation of normal bowel function. Other symptoms such as lethargy, malaise and headache, which are attributed to constipation by the patient should be treated on their merits. *They are often due to depression.*

(2) Attempts should also be made to re-educate the bowel. Following withdrawal of the stimulant laxative it is almost invariably necessary to replace it initially with an osmotic purgative such as magnesium or sodium sulphate. Increasing dietary fibre with bran and products such as Normacol, Isogel and Metamucil are also important. The patient must be warned that it is likely to take several months for treatment to prove effective. Many will not persevere and return to their previous stimulant laxative abuse. In the elderly there is less chance of successful conversion to the new regimen and it is often necessary for them to continue with stimulant laxatives.

In extremely rare cases the colon becomes totally unresponsive to increasing doses of purgatives. Colectomy and ileorectal anastomosis may then be necessary.

### Problems with specific laxatives

Some specific laxatives are associated with special problems.

*Liquid paraffin,* which acts as a lubricant laxative, may, in large doses, impair absorption of the fat soluble vitamins, A, D and K. In old people it may seep through a lax anal sphincter, causing soiling and pruritis ani. Aspiration pneumonitis, due to accidental inhalation, is another problem. It is particularly likely to occur in the elderly and debilitated or in the presence of oesophageal reflux, stricture or achalasia.

*Surfactant laxatives* such as dioctyl sodium sulphosuccinate and poloxalkol, which are constituents of Dulcodos and Dorbanex respectively, act by enhancing water penetration into stool. Recent evidence suggests they may interfere with small bowel absorption of concurrently taken drugs.

*Osmotic laxatives* are 'non-absorbable' compounds of sodium and magnesium. They are the major constituent of 'health salts'. By osmotic attraction they prevent absorption of water by the intestine which increases the fluidity of stool. Magnesium salts may also work by releasing cholecystokinin from the upper small intestine which, itself, affects colonic muscle activity. Over usage may cause electrolyte and fluid depletion. Although the majority of magnesium is not absorbed, small amounts do cross the intestinal mucosa. These are excreted in the urine, but in patients with renal impairment hypermagnesaemia with muscle weakness and confusion may occur.

*Bulk laxative* agents are non-absorbable, hydrophilic vegetable fibres. They stimulate bowel action mainly by virtue of their bulk, and because they retain water the stool remains soft and manageable. They are the safest of the laxative preparations but should be avoided in patients with oesophageal or bowel strictures.

*Stimulant laxatives* (anthraquinones, polyphenols and castor oil) are drugs which stimulate bowel peristalsis by direct action on the mucosa. They have a toxic effect on the myenteric plexus and may cause severe metabolic disturbance when used in excess over long periods.

Two drugs in this group cause specific problems. *Phenolphthalein* may induce skin irritation and rash which particularly affects the buttocks. *Oxyphenisatin* is contained in proprietary aperients available in Continental Europe but not in the United Kingdom. There is good evidence that it can cause a chronic active hepatitis.

## Differential diagnosis of constipation

Before assuming a diagnosis of 'simple' constipation the following disorders should be considered and eliminated.

*Carcinoma of the left side of the colon* or *rectosigmoid junction* may cause increasing constipation. The history is relatively short and there may be accompanying anorexia and weight loss. Blood may be noticed in the stool. Sigmoid tumours are often extrinsically palpable on rectal examination and visible with the sigmoidoscope. A double contrast barium enema will be necessary to exclude lesions beyond the range of the sigmoidoscope. *Strictures* resulting from *large bowel diverticulitis* and occasionally *colonic Crohn's disease* may also cause constipation. The history, barium enema and, when necessary, colonoscopy usually make the diagnosis clear.

*Depression* may often be accompanied by constipation but it is rarely the dominant presenting feature. *Hypothyroidism, hyperparathyroidism* and other causes of *hypercalcaemia* may cause constipation. Associated features of these disorders are almost invariably present.

It is essential to review *drug regimens* in those complaining of constipation. Antacids containing aluminium compounds and codeine-based cough linctuses are the commonest offenders.

137

Other drugs less often implicated are anticholinergics and methyldopa.

*Disease of the spinal cord or sacral nerve roots* may cause constipation and rectal loading. There is nearly always accompanying bladder dysfunction, together with neurological symptoms and signs in the legs. *Hirschsprung's disease,* which is caused by an aganglionic segment in the distal bowel, is a cause of severe constipation and gross colonic distension in infants. A few, relatively mild cases, have apparently not presented until adult life but this must be extremely rare.

## OTHER PROBLEMS WITH DEFAECATION

### Alternating diarrhoea and constipation

The three main causes are the *irritable bowel syndrome, purgative abuse* and *carcinoma of the left colon* or *rectosigmoid junction*.

An erratic bowel habit is most commonly due to the irritable bowel syndrome. The history usually distinguishes it from laxative abuse although purgation may be denied (see also Chapter 13). Alternating diarrhoea and constipation of recent onset should always raise the suspicion of carcinoma in the left side of the colon or rectosigmoid junction. It is especially likely if there is accompanying weight loss, anorexia or blood loss per rectum. Sigmoidoscopy and barium enema are essential when these symptoms present.

### Sensation of incomplete rectal emptying

Because *carcinoma of the rectum* often presents with this symptom, rectal examination and sigmoidoscopy are mandatory in such patients. Inflammatory conditions of the rectum, such as *ulcerative proctocolitis* and *Crohn's disease,* may also cause this sensation. The diagnosis is again made by sigmoidoscopy and rectal biopsy.

The *descending perineum syndrome* is characterized by a recurrent or continuous sensation of needing to defaecate. In this condition the anterior rectal mucosa prolapses which causes a sensation of something in the lumen of the anus. Further straining only produces more prolapse. There is probably an underlying disorder of anorectal muscle function. Sigmoidoscopy will often reveal a small patch of 'proctitis' on the anterior rectal wall in the vicinity of the rectal valve. Treatment consists of explanation and reassurance. The patient must be discouraged from straining and any coexistent constipation treated. *Solitary ulcer* of the anterior rectum appears to be a long term complication of the descending perineum syndrome. Patients with this condition are often obsessed by their bowel habit and frequently admit to digitally removing stool from the rectum. Sigmoidoscopy and biopsy distinguishes the ulcer from cancer. Treatment is unsatisfactory. When conservative measures fail some surgeons will attempt correction of the underlying prolapse.

The sensation of incomplete emptying may also occur in association with other symptoms in the *irritable bowel syndrome*. The usual complaint is that within minutes of passing stool the sensation to defaecate returns. Attempts to do so, however, results only in the passage of a few tiny pellet or thread like stools. Increasing the bulk of the stool with additional dietary fibre is often very helpful.

## Proctalgia fugax

This term is used to describe sudden severe pain in the perineum and rectum. It may occur spontaneously, or be precipitated by straining at stool and sexual intercourse. Nocturnal attacks are not uncommon. It lasts only a few seconds or minutes. The mechanism is not clear but probably results from spasm in the muscles of the pelvic floor or rectum.

In those patients whose symptoms are brought on by straining at stool, treatment includes relief of constipation. Pressure over the coccyx sometimes helps during an attack but there is otherwise no specific therapy. In patients experiencing frequent nocturnal attacks, or in those where sexual intercourse commonly precipitates the problem, diazepam is sometimes a useful prophylaxis. With reassurance most patients are able to tolerate their symptoms because the episodes are both infrequent and brief.

---

Recent onset of constipation in patients over 40 requires early investigation by sigmoidoscopy and barium enema to exclude colorectal cancer

---

# 17

# Miscellaneous Gastrointestinal Problems

## ANOREXIA

This symptom may be differentiated into (1) a true loss of appetite and (2) reduction of intake due to the precipitation of pain or other unpleasant symptoms. True loss of appetite occurs in debilitating conditions such as *malignant disease*, especially carcinoma of the stomach. It may be the presenting symptom in *pernicious anaemia* and frequently occurs in *uraemia, liver failure, tuberculosis, Crohn's disease* and *infectious hepatitis*.

Restriction of food intake due to the precipitation of pain occurs most commonly with *peptic ulcers,* or less commonly in *gastritis* and *reflux oesophagitis*. It is also found in *mesenteric angina, pancreatitis* and the *irritable bowel syndrome*.

Psychological factors are often important causes of anorexia. *Severe depression*, especially pathological grief, may be accompanied by a total loss of appetite. *Anorexia nervosa* classically occurs in teenage girls who do not admit to anorexia. In fact they talk at length about their enjoyment of food, failing to say they only take minute quantities owing to fear of becoming overweight. A related syndrome which occurs in the same sex and age group is bulimia nervosa, where the patient eats enormous quantities and then vomits the food up immediately. Both of these are accompanied by weight loss. It is an interesting fact that anorexia and nausea occur more frequently in *pregnancy* than do the traditionally accepted bizarre fads for certain foods.

## THE 'ABNORMAL' TONGUE

Patients present frequently at the surgery with what they believe is an abnormal tongue and can be quite obsessive about this, the symptoms often lasting for years in some cases. They may need repeated firm assurance. The two commonest complaints are changes in sensation and appearance. *Burning* or *tingling* is probably the most frequent complaint. In only one in five can a cause be found. This is usually due to deficiencies of iron, folic acid or the vitamin B complex including $B_{12}$ when the tongue becomes red and often painful. There may be a history of heavy pipe or cigarette smoking, recent antibiotic treatment or dental disorders. In the great majority no abnormality is found and firm reassurance, particularly regarding cancer, is necessary. The commonest complaint about the appearance of the tongue is coating. *A white or yellow* coating is a physiological phenomenon. It consists of desquamated epithelium, food debris and bacteria. It is most noticeable first thing in the morning and encouraged by smoking, mouth-breathing and fasting. The latter two causes are the likely explanation of the furred tongue seen in a pyrexial patient. A *black hairy* tongue is thought to be due to bacterial or fungal proliferation, particularly after antibiotic therapy. It is quite harmless, resolves spontaneously and, like physiological coating requires no specific treatment. Scrubbing the tongue and powerful mouthwashes should be avoided.

*Fissuring, the geographical tongue,* and the discovery of the large *circumvallate papillae* at the back of the tongue are often cause for 'alarm'. Strong reassurance is usually all that is needed.

*Aphthous ulcers* affect the tongue and the buccal mucosa. General debility, emotional stress and local irritation may be cited as aetiological factors, but association with other diseases is non-specific. Healing is spontaneous and topical steroids, carbenoxolone and disodium chromoglycate have never been shown consistently to enhance healing.

In a few patients examination reveals disease requiring investigation and definitive treatment. These include *carcinomatous* and *syphilitic lesions, leukoplakia* and *macroglossia* due to *amyloidosis* or *myxoedema*.

## BAD BREATH

Bad breath is a common complaint which should be differentiated into that which is obvious to other people and that of which only the patient is aware. The latter is often combined with a bad taste in the mouth and is usually part of an obsessional neurosis. A thorough examination, reassurance and the encouragement not to indulge in excessive oral toilet is helpful, but reassurance may have to be repeated. Rarely, a psychiatric opinion may be necessary. Halitosis on waking is normal and likely to be more severe in mouth-breathers and smokers. Having breakfast and cleaning the teeth usually solve the problem. Dental and gingival disease together with poor oral hygiene cause day-long halitosis, as can frequent indulgence in eating garlic and onions. Occasionally animal fats and meat proteins can cause bad breath due to volatile metabolic products and restriction of these in the diet is worth trying.

Chronic sepsis and neoplasia of the nasopharynx can cause an unpleasant odour, but is usually a comparatively insignificant symptom. The classic foetors of ketosis, uraemia and hepatic failure, while helpful in making a diagnosis, are rarely complained of by the patient. *Bad breath is not an indication of a bowel disease or the result of constipation.*

## WIND AND GASEOUSNESS

'Excessive gas' in the alimentary tract is a common complaint. The most frequent symptoms are belching, excessive flatus, colic, borborygmi and the feeling of abdominal distension without being able to obtain relief.

Ninety-nine per cent of the gas in the alimentary tract is composed of oxygen, carbon dioxide, nitrogen, hydrogen and methane. Swallowed air is the major source of oxygen and nitrogen. Bacteria produce hydrogen and methane. Carbon dioxide is mainly endogenous, being produced by bacterial fermentation and the acidification of bicarbonate-containing secretions. Small amounts of highly odiferous gases produced by colonic bacteria make up the remaining 1%.

Excessive gas production is a feature of certain specific disorders. *Small bowel diverticulosis* leads to bacterial proliferation, while *small intestinal malabsorption* and *maldigestion* due to pancreatic disease results in an increased substrate for colonic bacteria. Treating the underlying condition is the key to successful management. In the great majority of patients, however, no underlying cause is evident. No appreciable gas is produced in the stomach except in *pyloric stenosis and therefore patients whose main complaint is belching almost invariably practice aerophagy.* This is often a feature of *anxiety.* It is also practised by patients suffering from oesophagitis who continually swallow saliva to neutralize the irritant gastric acid which has refluxed into the distal oesophagus. *Chewing gum, eating and drinking too quickly* and *irritant mouth lesions* can encourage air ingestion. Most of this is belched but some passes distally contributing to the feeling of distension. Patients who complain of *abdominal distension and pain* have been shown experimentally to have *no excess of gastrointestinal gas.* The main problem is the inability to accommodate normal volumes without pain. The patients often have a very slow transit time through the gut and gas tends to collect in the hepatic and splenic flexures. Gaseousness is a common complaint in the *irritable bowel syndrome*.

The curing of belching thus depends on treating the underlying anxiety and correcting any factors encouraging aerophagy. This also applies to patients complaining of pain, borborygmi and abdominal distension. The basic pathogenic mechanism does not appear to be excessive production of gas, but measures to reduce flatus formation should be attempted. Dietary manipulation is helpful. It is accepted that cabbage and beans have an inflationary effect, but it is less well known that apple and grape juice, raisins and bananas also encourage gas formation (*see* Appendix, low flatulence diet and low residue diet). Attempts to alleviate symptoms by changing bacterial flora with antibiotics have not had consistent success and similar claims for charcoal, kaolin and chlorophyll have not been substantiated.

## ANAL IRRITATION

Anal irritation is a common problem which is often dealt with by the patient in a variety of ways, frequently making the problem much worse by the time he or she presents at the surgery. It is most commonly caused by the lack of efficient perianal cleansing. Faeces lurk in the furrowed skin and combined with moisture serve to break down the normal resistance of the skin. The irritation set up leads to scratching and this abrades the surface. Once the surface layer is breached it becomes host to bacteria and fungi. At this point the patient will apply lotions, ointments and creams usually recommended by friends or chemists. Some of these may damage the area further, producing an eczema-like rash.

The irritation can be removed by following a few basic principles. Initially *thorough gentle washing* after every bowel action and night and morning, using a bidet or handshower preferably, though a bowl of water will do. Soap should be used sparingly. The skin should be dried gently by dabbing. It should be kept dry throughout the day. A pledget of cotton wool dusted with drying powder, e.g. Zeasorb, can be kept against the anus. Avoid nylon underwear and wear loose fitting trousers or skirts. Tights should not be worn. Avoid perfumed talcum powder which may cause an allergy and greasy ointments which may make the skin soggy. A 50% solution of magenta paint in water is a useful antiseptic drying lotion. Foods which cause anal irritation or looseness should be avoided and bowels should be opened regularly without straining. Constipation is best treated by smooth bulk-forming aperients such as fibre supplements. Aggravating conditions such as haemorrhoids and fungal infections should be dealt with concurrently.

# 18
# Jaundice and Common Liver Diseases

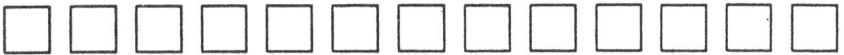

Jaundice occurs when the total bilirubin level in the serum rises above 2 mg per 100 ml. It may be classified pathophysiologically into the following categories:

haemolysis
dyserythropoiesis
non-haemolytic hyperbilirubinaemias
hepatocellular
extra- and intrahepatic cholestasis

However, when faced with a jaundiced patient it is simpler to consider the common causes of jaundice and by using clinical, laboratory and imaging information the diagnosis can be readily achieved in the majority of cases. An appropriate referral for medical or surgical management can then be made.

## DIAGNOSIS

### Unconjugated hyperbilirubinaemia

Raised levels of unconjugated bilirubin are the characteristic of the jaundice in haemolytic disease, dyserythropoiesis, the commonest cause of which is pernicious anaemia, and the non-haemolytic hyperbilirubinaemias. *Bilirubinuria is not found in these disorders* because unconjugated bilirubin is not passed in the urine. This contrasts with cholestatic and hepatocellular disease in which bilirubinuria occurs.

## Haemolytic and dyserythropoietic disease

In these conditions jaundice only occurs when the liver's capacity to metabolize haem is swamped. This occurs uncommonly and jaundice is rarely a dominant feature of these disorders. They are easily distinguished from hepatocellular and cholestatic disease by:

(1) the accompanying anaemia,
(2) a reticulocytosis,
(3) the blood film and bone marrow,
(4) absence of bile in the urine.

## Non-haemolytic unconjugated hyperbilirubinaemia

The only disease in this category likely to be commonly encountered in general practice is *Gilbert's disease*. This is an inherited disorder and is probably transmitted by an autosomal dominant mechanism. Jaundice is due to a deficiency of the hepatic enzyme UDP glucuronyl transferase which is necessary for the efficient conversion of unconjugated bilirubin to the conjugated form. It is only the conjugated form that can be excreted in bile and therefore the levels of unconjugated bilirubin rise in the serum. A significant deficiency of the enzyme is present in approximately 5% of the British population, but clinically apparent icterus from this disorder is rare. Jaundice can be precipitated or exacerbated in Gilbert's disease by starvation. Anorexia induced by any illness may, therefore, be accompanied by mild jaundice in those with Gilbert's disease. A a consequence there is sometimes confusion with viral hepatitis. The two conditions are easily distinguished because in Gilbert's disease the serum alkaline phosphatase and transaminase levels are normal and there is no bile in the urine.

### Hepatocellular and cholestatic jaundice

The majority of patients with jaundice have either hepatocellular or cholestatic disease. The commonest of these and the main mechanism for the jaundice are:

| | |
|---|---|
| Viral hepatitis | – hepatocellular |
| Alcoholic hepatitis | – hepatocellular |
| Drugs | – hepatocellular or intrahepatic cholestasis |
| Gallstones | – extrahepatic cholestasis |
| Carcinoma of pancreas | – extrahepatic cholestasis |

| | |
|---|---|
| Secondary hepatic carcinoma | – intrahepatic and extrahepatic cholestasis |
| Chronic hepatitis | – hepatocellular |
| Primary biliary cirrhosis | – intrahepatic cholestasis |
| Cirrhosis | – hepatocellular and intrahepatic cholestasis |

alcoholic
auto-immune
hepatitis B
cryptogenic

## Associated clinical features

In hepatocellular and cholestatic jaundice, associated clinical features are frequently helpful pointers towards a diagnosis. The commonest are:

| | |
|---|---|
| Acute anorexia and nausea | – viral hepatitis |
| Chronic anorexia and weight loss | – malignant disease |
| Chronic lethargy and malaise | – malignant disease or cirrhosis |
| Diarrhoea | – chronic liver disease complicating inflammatory bowel disease |
| Pale stool and dark urine | – any severe hepatocellular disease or cholestatic disease |
| Modest pyrexia | – viral hepatitis |
| Severe pyrexia/rigors | – cholangitis due to obstruction of extrahepatic ducts |
| Pain | |
| epigastric and severe | – biliary colic due to stone |
| epigastric and continuous often radiating to the back | – carcinoma of pancreas |
| right hypochondrial | – hepatitis – viral or alcoholic |
| Pruritis | – usually due to cholestasis resulting from: extrahepatic obstruction, drug-induced cholestasis, primary |

147

|                                    |   |                                                                       |
|------------------------------------|---|-----------------------------------------------------------------------|
|                                    |   | biliary cirrhosis, cholestatic phase of viral hepatitis               |
| Rash                               | – | viral illness; glandular fever, hepatitis B                           |
| Arthritis                          | – | hepatitis B                                                           |
| Drugs<br>  therapeutic             | – | most commonly involved are:<br>   isoniazid<br>   methyldopa<br>   chlorpromazine and other phenothiazines<br>   chlorpropamide<br>   nitrofurantoin<br>   azathioprine<br>   17-alkylated steroids<br>   contraceptive pill<br>   oxyphenisatin |
|   overdose                         | – | paracetamol                                                           |
|   anaesthetic                      | – | halothane, especially after repeated exposure                         |
| Chemical exposure                  | – | aromatic solvents                                                     |
| Alcohol                            | – | chronic abuse; cirrhosis, alcoholic hepatitis                         |
|                                    | – | binge; alcoholic hepatitis, pancreatitis causing bile duct obstruction |
| Surgery                            | – | previous cholecystectomy, consider retained stone or bile duct stricture |
| Infusion of blood products         | – | non-A, non-B hepatitis                                                |
| Contaminated needles               | – | recent tattooing, drug addiction – hepatitis B                        |
| Sexual contact                     | – | hepatitis B, especially male homosexuals                              |
| Oedema and ascites                 | – | uncompensated cirrhosis or secondary carcinoma                        |
| Cutaneous signs (clubbing, white nails, bruising, spider naevi, palmar erythema) | – | cirrhosis, chronic active hepatitis |

148

| | | |
|---|---|---|
| Xanthoma | – | primary biliary cirrhosis |
| Gynaecomastia and testicular atrophy | – | cirrhosis, chronic active hepatitis, alcoholic hepatitis |
| Parotid enlargement and Dupuytren's contracture | – | alcoholic liver disease |
| Lymphadenopathy | – | malignant disease |
| Hepatomegaly | | |
| smooth edge | – | alcoholic liver disease |
| tender | – | alcoholic and viral hepatitis, or congestive cardiac failure |
| hard and irregular | – | secondary carcinoma or macronodular cirrhosis |
| Palpable gall bladder | – | carcinoma of pancreas |
| Splenomegaly and distended abdominal veins | – | portal hypertension usually due to cirrhosis |

## INVESTIGATION

### Initial tests

Standard liver function tests are of limited value in identifying the cause of jaundice. However, the following are helpful guidelines:

| | | |
|---|---|---|
| Serum bilirubin | – | variable in hepatitis and chronic liver disease |
| | – | highest levels found in common bile duct obstruction (cancer of pancreas and stone) |
| Alkaline phosphatase | – | usually modest in viral or alcoholic hepatitis |
| | – | very high in: pancreatic carcinoma, common bile duct stone, secondary carcinoma and advanced primary biliary cirrhosis |
| Serum transaminases | – | very high (more than 1000 iu) in acute hepatitis |
| | – | modest in chronic hepatitis and cirrhosis |
| | – | slight elevation or normal in biliary obstruction |

149

| | |
|---|---|
| Serum γ-glutamyl transpeptidase | – usually reflect alkaline phosphate levels |
| | – when high and other enzymes normal, alcoholic liver disease is probable |
| Plasma proteins | – low albumin: chronic liver disease |
| | – raised globulins: chronic hepatitis |
| Urine tests | – bilirubinuria *present* in hepatocellular or cholestatic disease; *absent* in unconjugated bilirubinaemias |
| | – urobilinogen absent with complete bile duct obstruction |
| Viral serology | – tests available for identifying hepatitis A, hepatitis B, glandular fever and cytomegalovirus |
| Autoantibodies | – mitrochondrial antibody + in primary biliary cirrhosis |
| | – smooth muscle antibody + in auto-immune chronic hepatitis |

## Further investigation

In many instances more invasive investigation is required to achieve a diagnosis.

### Chest X-ray and GI endoscopy

If clinical evidence suggests secondary carcinoma, chest X-ray and endoscopic examination of the stomach may rapidly achieve a diagnosis.

### Percutaneous liver biopsy

When the clinical and biochemical features indicate viral hepatitis further investigation is unnecessary. However, if jaundice persists or liver function tests fail to improve within 6 months of suggested viral hepatitis, liver biopsy should be obtained. This will enable distinction between chronic persistent hepatitis, which does not require specific treatment and chronic active hepatitis which does.

Liver biopsy is also helpful in confirming suspected drug-induced jaundice. In the alcoholic abuser, severity of liver damage can be identified and a more accurate prognosis obtained. Micronodular cirrhosis can be diagnosed with accuracy by percutaneous needle biopsy because the abnormality tends to be diffuse. In contrast, macronodular cirrhosis may be missed by this technique as there are often large areas of liver where normal architecture is preserved. Histology of the liver will also separate jaundice due principally to hepatocellular disease from cholestatic conditions. In this latter group it is usually possible to distinguish primary biliary cirrhosis from other causes, but it is not always possible for the histopathologists to separate other causes of intrahepatic cholestasis from extrahepatic obstruction.

## Laparoscopy

Laparoscopy can be performed following intravenous diazepam and local anaesthesia of the anterior abdominal wall. The hepatic surface can be inspected and biopsies of specific areas obtained under direct vision. It is therefore of particular value when carcinomatosis or macronodular cirrhosis is suspected.

## Radio-isotope scanning

In cirrhosis, radio-isotopes are taken up poorly by the liver, whereas the spleen has an increased avidity for the isotope. The technique is also useful for the detection of primary and secondary hepatic carcinomatous deposits.

## Ultrasound screening

The increased sophistication of ultrasonic scanning has been a major advance in the management of jaundice. The principal benefit of ultrasound is its ability to detect dilated intra- and extrahepatic bile ducts. This enables patients with jaundice to be readily divided into those with an obstructive lesion of the large bile ducts, potentially amenable to surgery, and those with other causes who do not require laparotomy. In addition, ultrasonic scanning may show the cause of obstruction, which is most commonly gallstone or carcinoma of the pancreas. When dilated ducts are not found, this usually indicates an hepatic cause of jaundice and in these circumstances an experienced observer can usually distinguish cirrhosis from other pathologies.

## Cholangiography

The routine oral cholecystogram and intravenous cholangiogram are of no use in the presence of hepatocellular and cholestatic jaundice because the radio-opaque medium is not secreted in sufficient concentration. There are two principal alternatives that can be used to demonstrate the biliary system.

## Endoscopic retrograde cholangiopancreatography (ERCP)

This involves the passage of a fine catheter through the biopsy channel of a flexible upper gastrointestinal endoscope into the ampulla of Vater. A radio-opaque medium is then injected into the biliary system. It will confirm or exclude dilation and obstruction of the biliary ducts. This technique has two additional benefits. One is that the pancreatic ducts can also be examined, which may reveal pancreatitis or carcinoma. The second advantage is the facility to remove stones from the common bile duct and introduce drainage stents without the need for laparotomy.

## Percutaneous transhepatic cholangiography (PTC)

This involves the passage of a very fine flexible needle through anaesthetized skin into the liver. When a bile duct is located, radio-opaque medium is injected which demonstrates either a dilated or normal biliary system. Patients in the former category are then referred for early surgery. The major advantage of this technique over ERCP is its relative simplicity, but it does not, of course, demonstrate the pancreatic ducts. In addition there is no facility for removal of stones, but a modification of the method does allow a flexible drainage catheter to be percutaneously positioned in the liver so that jaundice can be temporarily relieved.

The diagnostic investigation is schematized in Figure 18.1.

## MANAGEMENT OF SOME SPECIFIC LIVER DISEASES

### Viral hepatitis

Three distinct categories of viral hepatitis are now recognized. They are type A, type B and type non-A, non-B. This last group almost certainly includes several different, as yet unidentified, organisms.

### Type A

This disease can now be confirmed by the finding of specific serum IgM antibodies to the virus.

Admission to hospital is not necessary in most cases. The patient usually confines himself to bed during the first few days but as soon as he begins to improve strict bed rest is not essential. Barrier nursing is unnecessary but the patient must exercise special care with the disposal of excreta and washing of hands for at least a week after the appearance of jaundice. Use of a separate lavatory is ideal. A free diet should be allowed. *Drugs, including cortico-*

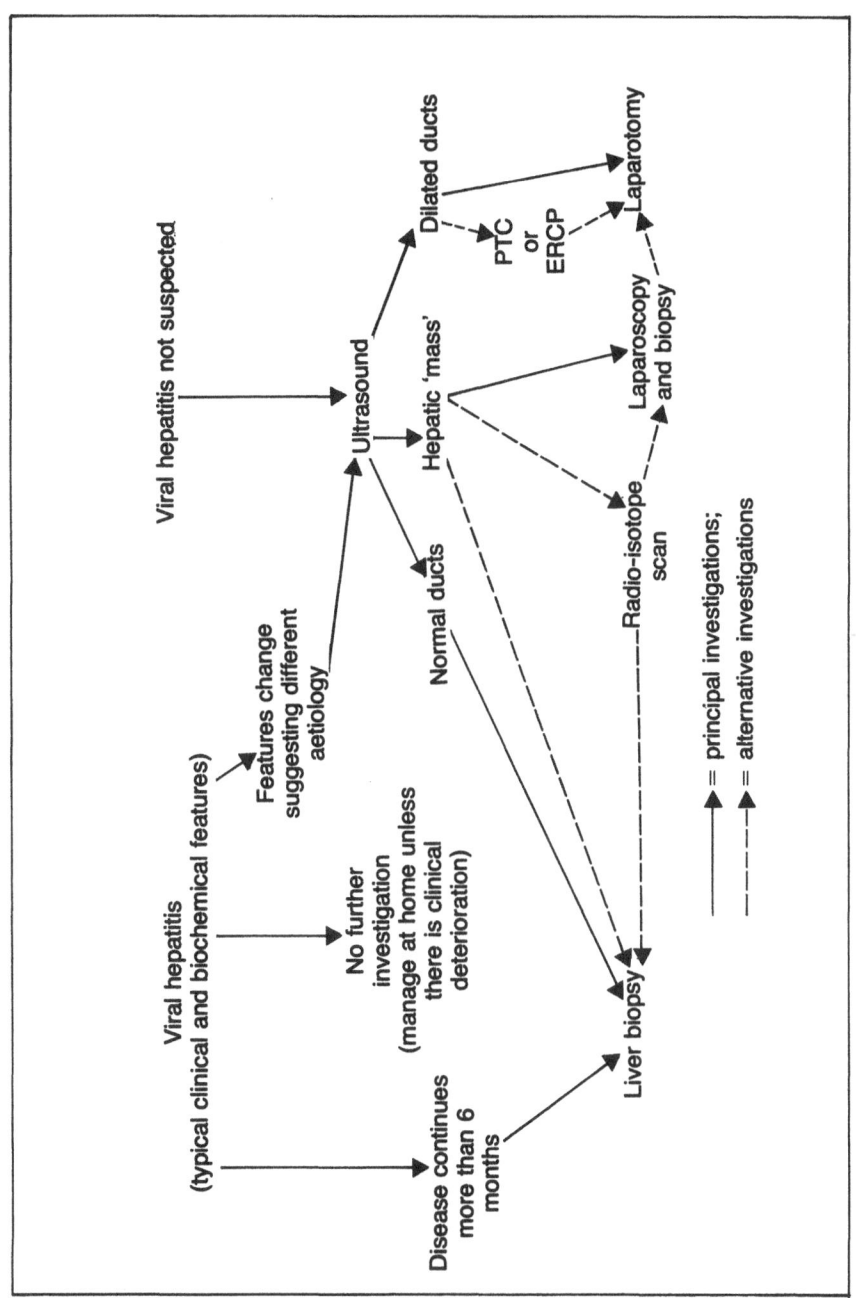

**Figure 18.1**  Diagnostic investigation of hepatocellular and cholestatic jaundice

*steroids, are of no proven benefit in the routine management of acute viral hepatitis. Six months abstinence from alcohol is obligatory.*

*Admission to hospital.* Admission to hospital is usually for social reasons which include unsatisfactory toilet arrangements, absence of someone to look after the patient or the presence of infants in the house. The other major reason for admission is the severity of the disease (*see below,* Fulminant hepatitis).

*Prevention.* Travellers to countries with a high incidence of hepatitis may be protected for 2 months by a prophylactic intramuscular injection of human γ-globulin. This is also effective in preventing the disease in contacts of hepatitis patients when given within 2 weeks of exposure.

## Type B

The principles of management are the same as those for hepatitis A and admission to hospital is governed by the same factors.

*Prevention.* The serum of patients should be monitored to ensure that they have not developed chronic hepatitis or become carriers of the virus. A specific antihepatitis B immunoglobulin is available. When contaminated material is accidentally introduced, either by splashing on to mucous membranes or by pricking, the specific immunoglobulin should be administered as soon as possible and repeated at 4 weeks. *The sexual partners of patients should also be offered prophylaxis.* Vaccination against hepatitis B virus is now available, but is at present reserved for those at high risk such as hospital personnel and sexual partners of certain antigen-positive patients.

## Type non-A, non-B

This agent appears to be an important cause of hepatitis transmitted by blood products, although it can also be spread by the non-parenteral route. The incubation period varies from 5 weeks to 5 months. It is a probable cause of chronic liver disease. Management is as described for type D hepatitis, but as yet there are no specific serological markers of the disease or vaccines available.

## Complications of viral hepatitis

Viral hepatitis may be complicated by:

(1)   fulminant hepatitis
(2)   prolonged cholestasis
(3)   chronic hepatitis

154

(4) cirrhosis

(5) hepatoma

*Fulminant hepatitis*. Fortunately, fulminant hepatitis is very rare. In a few cases of rapidly progressive hepatitis the patient's condition deteriorates before the jaundice has fully developed. More commonly, a fulminant course is accompanied by deepening jaundice, and in such cases admission to hospital is clearly vital. Other ominous features are vomiting, bruising and signs of encephalopathy, including a flapping tremor, confusion, stupor or coma.

*Prolonged cholestasis*. In a minority of patients jaundice fails to resolve within the usual 4–6 weeks, despite an obvious general improvement. Itching becomes troublesome and the liver function tests have a cholestatic pattern with greatly elevated levels of alkaline phosphatase and a comparatively small rise in the transaminases. The condition must be distinguished from extrahepatic biliary obstruction and drug jaundice. The condition resolves clinically and histologically within 6 months.

*Chronic hepatitis*. Chronic hepatitis can be defined as inflammation of the liver which continues for more than 6 months without evidence of resolution. it is a sequel to type B and probably type non-A,non-B infection (*see below,* Chronic Hepatitis).

*Cirrhosis*. The discovery of serological markers for hepatitis B infection has confirmed that infection with this virus may, in a small proportion of patients, progress to cirrhosis.

*Hepatoma*. There is a high incidence of primary hepatocellular cancer in areas of the world where hepatitis B infection is common. Although cirrhosis and hepatoma are closely associated, the former is not always present in patients with type B serological markers and hepatoma, which suggests that the virus may be directly oncogenic.

## Chronic hepatitis

Chronic hepatitis is defined as inflammation of the liver which continues for more than 6 months without evidence of resolution. Two distinct categories, largely based upon histological features, are recognized. They are chronic persistent and chronic active hepatitis.

### Chronic persistent hepatitis

The histological characteristics of chronic persistent hepatitis are mononuclear cell infiltration of the portal tracts, preservation of normal lobular structure and absence of 'piecemeal' necrosis. *The diagnosis can only be made with certainty by liver biopsy.*

Although many causes of chronic persistent hepatitis have been identified the aetiology is obscure in many cases. *Hepatitis types B* and *non-A,non-B* may persist for more than 6 months. An acute *alcoholic hepatitis* may progress in similar fashion. *Ulcerative colitis, Crohn's* and *coeliac disease* may also be associated with these histological features in the liver. *Drugs,* including paracetamol, aspirin, methyldopa, isoniazid and some cytotoxic agents are capable of inducing a persistent hepatic inflammatory reaction.

There is no specific treatment and steroids are not indicated. Prolonged abstinence from alcohol is essential. Although the patient must be warned that recovery may take several years, he should be strongly reassured that it will be complete and that cirrhosis will not develop.

## Chronic active hepatitis

The histological characteristics of this condition are lymphocyte and plasma cell infiltration of the portal tracts, disruption of the liver lobule with 'piecemeal' necrosis and extensive fibrosis.

As with chronic persistent hepatitis, *types B* and *non-A,non-B viruses, alcohol* and *drugs* (oxyphenisatin, methyldopa, isoniazid) are known aetiological agents. The majority of cases have no known cause. Within this latter group are those patients with *lupoid hepatitis,* which is characterized by an association with auto-immune phenomena and other autoallergic diseases. When chronic active hepatitis occurs in children or adolescents, *Wilson's disease* must also be considered. This condition is due to a metabolic defect which leads to copper deposition in body tissues. The areas most severely affected are the basal ganglia and liver. It is an inherited condition and the mode of transmission is autosomal recessive. Consanguinity of patients is found in more than 50% of cases.

The pathogenic processes in chronic active hepatitis are not understood but it has been suggested that viruses, drugs, alcohol and probably other agents initiate liver damage. This releases or changes the antigenicity of liver tissue which, in turn, stimulates an auto-immune process. Clones of lymphocytes sensitized in this way then continue damaging the liver in the absence of the initiating agent. It seems likely that affected subjects have a genetic predisposition to mount inappropriate immune reactions.

*When a cause can be identified the following courses of management should be adopted.*

*Drug induced disease.* The offending drug must be withdrawn and should not be reintroduced. Under these circumstances the disease is not progressive and prognosis is good.

*Wilson's disease*. Continuing liver damage can be arrested by early treatment with the chelating agent, penicillamine. Prognosis is comparatively good in those treated before neurological symptoms have appeared. Untreated, the liver lesion progresses. The common causes of death are hepatocellular failure, haemorrhage from varices or one of the complications of severe neurological deficit.

*Lupoid hepatitis*. Prednisolone 10 – 15 mg daily leads to clinical, biochemical and histological improvement in a large proportion of patients and early mortality is reduced. Treatment should continue for at least 6 months and may be needed for several years in some cases. Azathioprine 50 mg daily is sometimes added to the prednisolone regime, particularly in those who fail to respond to the steroid alone. The natural progression of the liver lesion is to cirrhosis. Without treatment there is a 60% mortality within 5 years of onset from either liver failure or bleeding varices. The effect of treatment on long term survival is not yet clear.

*Virus type B chronic active hepatitis*. The value of prednisolone and azathioprine in this group has yet to be proved. However, in patients with significant symptoms Sherlock suggests a 6-month trial of prednisolone 10 – 20 mg daily, the benefit being assessed clinically, biochemically and histologically. If there is no obvious improvement it is unlikely that a more prolonged course will be useful. In patients with only minor symptoms steroid therapy is probably not indicated. However, if rebiopsy at 6 months indicates progression of the hepatic lesion, it seems reasonable to give a trial course of prednisolone. In general, this type of chronic active hepatitis progresses towards cirrhosis more slowly than lupoid hepatitis. There is, however, an increased risk of primary liver cell carcinoma.

## Drug-induced hepatic dysfunction

There is no specific therapy in most instances and all that is necessary is to withdraw the offending agent. Even when there is no conclusive proof that the suspected drug is the cause it should be stopped. Proof that it was involved is provided by resolution of the liver disturbance although this may take many months. The drug or its close relatives should not be given again. The notes must be clearly marked to avoid accidental readministration and the patient should wear an appropriate warning bracelet.

## Cirrhosis

The common causes of cirrhosis are:

(1)   type B and type non-A, non-B virus hepatitis,
(2)   chronic active hepatitis of any aetiology (see above),
(3)   alcohol,
(4)   persisting cholestasis (extrahepatic biliary obstruction or primary biliary cirrhosis)

More rarely it may be the result of longstanding severe cardiac failure. This is most likely to occur when the failure is predominantly right-sided or due to constrictive pericarditis. Deposition of substances such as iron in *haemochromatosis* and copper in *Wilson's disease* are other rare causes of cirrhosis. In addition to those cases of known aetiology there are a significant number in which the cause is unknown. These are labelled *cryptogenic*. With advancing knowledge and more accurate diagnostic techniques the proportion in this category has decreased.

### *Specific measures*

There is no specific therapy for the great majority of patients with cirrhosis. There are three exceptions to this. *Haemochromatosis* is treated by repeated venesection to mobilize iron stored in the liver. *Wilson's disease* may be arrested by long term treatment with the chelating agent, penicillamine, which removes copper from the tissues and promotes its excretion in the urine. Prednisolone, with or without azathioprine, is used when there is an associated *chronic active hepatitis*.

### Compensated cirrhosis

In well-compensated cirrhosis no active treatment is required other than abstinence from alcohol and the eating of a normal diet.

### Decompensated cirrhosis

### *Ascites*

The formation of ascites is a sign of decompensation and results from a combination of hepatocellular failure and portal venous hypertension. It is a serious complication and when it occurs insidiously the prognosis is particularly poor. In contrast, ascites of sudden onset, which is often precipitated by an alcoholic binge or gastrointestinal haemorrhage, has a better prognosis providing the patient can be adequately supported during the acute phase.

Admission to hospital is usually necessary because the initial treatment requires close monitoring.

The mainstays of treatment are:

bed rest
sodium restriction
fluid restriction
cautious diuretic therapy

Therapeutic paracentesis of ascites in cirrhosis depletes the body's protein pool. The procedure is potentially dangerous because it may precipitate circulatory failure and encephalopathy. It is now very rarely performed in cirrhosis.

Recurrence of ascites is very common after discharge from hospital. This is usually due to dietary lapse; persistent encouragement to keep to a 'no added' salt regimen (40–60 mmol sodium/day) is therefore necessary. Close monitoring of electrolytes and urea is important in those on maintenance diuretics.

In rare cases with resistant ascites, when dietary restriction and diuretic therapy has failed, a LeVeen peritoneovenous shunt may be implanted. This allows drainage of ascitic fluid from the peritoneum to the internal jugular vein via a subcutaneously implanted synthetic tube.

### Encephalopathy

Encephalopathy may be acute or chronic.

*Acute encephalopathy*. There are two main objectives in the management of acute hepatic encephalopathy:

(1) identification and treatment of the precipitating factor; and

(2) general measures to alleviate the encephalopathy.

The common precipitating causes of encephalopathy in a previously compensated patient are:

inappropriate diuretic therapy,
gastrointestinal haemorrhage,
an alcoholic binge,
severe diarrhoea and vomiting from any cause,
infections, usually respiratory or urinary tract,
potent analgesics and sedatives,
surgery,
constipation,

159

too much dietary protein,
drainage of large volumes of ascitic fluid.

The general practitioner should be aware of the hazards of using morphine and related analgesics, sedatives and overenthusiastic diuretic therapy in patients with cirrhosis. The prompt treatment of infections and constipation will often prevent the development of encephalopathy.

*Nevertheless, it should be stressed that once there is evidence of impending encephalopathy or when the precipitating cause itself requires inpatient treatment, hospital admission should be arranged without delay.*

Treatment will include:

protein restriction,
adequate calories as carbohydrate,
oral neomycin,
lactulose,
purgation,
correction of hypokalaemia,
systemic antibiotics (infection is a common cause of decompensation).

*Chronic encephalopathy.* The neuropsychiatric features of chronic hepatic encephalopathy may be alleviated by restriction of dietary protein and long term use of lactulose or neomycin. Because some types of hepatic encephalopathy resemble parkinsonism in which brain dopamine is depleted, *laevodopa* has been used. Unfortunately, it has no lasting effect. *Bromocriptine,* a dopamine agonist, has also been tried, but further studies are required before it can be recommended for routine use. In resistant cases, *colectomy* or *colonic exclusion* operations have been employed as a means of reducing bacterial 'toxin' production. *Transplantation* of a donor liver has been of limited success in a few cases.

## Osteomalacia

The bone pain of osteomalacia can be successfully treated with intramuscular vitamin D 100 000 – 150 000 units weekly. The serum calcium and bone alkaline phosphatase levels must be monitored and a suitable maintenance dose found by trial in each patient.

## Loss of libido and impotence

This problem usually proves resistant to treatment. Nevertheless, testosterone orally or as a long acting intramuscular injection is worth trying.

---

Deterioration of mental function in a patient with cirrhosis is most commonly due to:

- inappropriate use of analgesics, sedatives and diuretics
- constipation
- infection
- gastrointestinal haemorrhage

---

*Hepatic ascites*

- Hepatic ascites is controlled by sodium and fluid restriction and diuretics
- Drainage of large volumes is dangerous

---

## Alcoholic liver disease

Disease of the liver due to alcohol can be divided into three main categories:

(1) fatty deposition (steatosis),
(2) hepatitis,
(3) cirrhosis.

Two thirds of all cases of cirrhosis in England and Wales are now due to alcohol. There are no diagnostic blood tests but the combination of an erythrocyte mean corpuscular volume greater than 100 c.microns and an elevated $\gamma$ -glutamyl transpeptidase should raise suspicion of alcohol related liver disease. Liver biopsy is the only definite means of diagnosing which category of disease is present and should be performed whenever liver dysfunction persists in those considered to be abusing alcohol.

### Advice to the patient

In patients whose biopsies show only fatty deposition and in whom there is no psychological dependence on alcohol, total abstinence may be unnecessary. Providing such patients keep consumption within reasonable limits it is unlikely they will develop more severe forms of alcoholic liver disease. It is impossible to be dogmatic about what is a reasonable amount, but two facts should be kept in mind: (1) women have a far greater risk of developing severe alcoholic liver disease and their 'safe amount' is less than for men, and (2) for men the daily consumption over a 10-year period of one third of a bottle of spirits or one bottle of table wine, or two thirds of a bottle of sherry or 5–6 pints (about 3–3.5 litres) of beer is associated with a high risk of alcoholic cirrhosis. Obviously patients must be instructed to keep well below these levels. Avoiding lunchtime drinking and restricting consumption to the evening will often force a heavy drinker into more acceptable and healthy habits.

In patients dependent upon alcohol, regardless of the degree of liver pathology, and in those with hepatitis, total abstinence is essential. This is necessary because there is overwhelming evidence that alcoholic hepatitis is a precirrhotic condition. In cirrhosis total abstinence seems also to prolong life significantly, especially in those patients who have not already suffered from variceal haemorrhage (Figure 18.2).

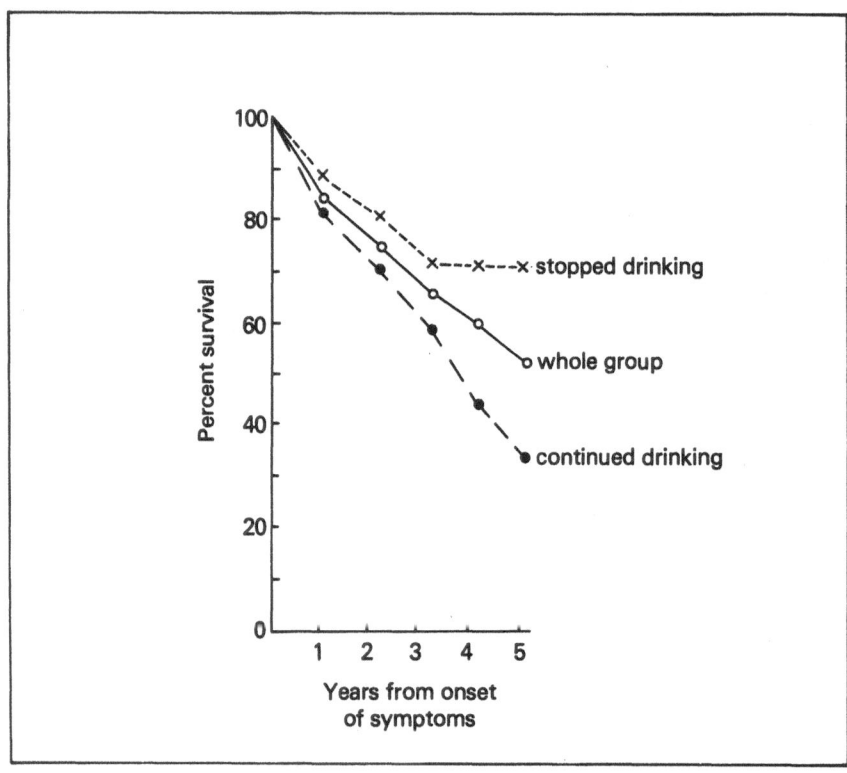

**Figure 18.2** Probability of survival in patients with alcoholic liver disease (from Lancaster-Smith, M. and Williams, K. (1982) *Problems in Gastroenterology*. (Lancaster: MTP Press))

### Additional measures

Alcohol dependence should be dealt with along the usual lines. Psychiatrists, social workers and self-help organizations, such as Alcoholics Anonymous, should be appropriately employed.

*Withdrawal of alcohol usually requires admission to hospital*. The severity of symptoms is alleviated by *chlormethiazol* (Heminevrin). This drug should not be continued for more than a few days because prolonged use may lead to dependency. High potency *vitamin B* should also be given parenterally to prevent a Wernicke–Korsakov syndrome. A *high protein* diet is desirable, providing hepatic encephalopathy is not induced.

There is no specific treatment for alcoholic steatosis or cirrhosis. The use of corticosteroids in alcoholic hepatitis is controversial. It should probably be reserved for severe cases. The recommended dose is prednisolone 40 mg daily for approximately 2 weeks.

### Prognosis

This is as follows.

(1) The prognosis in patients with fatty change alone is excellent, providing consumption of alcohol is controlled.

(2) Although steatosis is not a precirrhotic condition, continuance of heavy drinking will lead to hepatitis or cirrhosis in susceptible individuals.

(3) At present it is not possible to identify those at particular risk.

(4) The majority of patients with hepatitis who continue to drink will go on to cirrhosis.

(5) In general, alcoholic cirrhosis has a better prognosis than non-alcoholic cirrhosis.

(6) Approximate 5-year survival figures in alcoholic cirrhosis are 60% for abstainers and 40% for persisting drinkers.

# Appendix

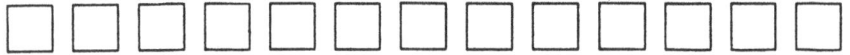

## INFORMATION FOR PATIENTS WITH GASTRO-OESOPHAGEAL REFLUX

Everybody's stomach occasionally forces some of its contents into the lower part of the gullet. This usually passes unnoticed but if it occurs continually symptoms will arise.

The commonest symptom is 'heartburn'. (In fact the problem has *nothing* to do with the heart.) The pain is usually described as 'burning' but other sensations are common, including 'sharp pains', and 'like a lump'. Sometimes gastric contents may actually come back into the mouth, and belching is very common.

Pain occurs because irritant substances in the gastric juices, especially acid, cause irritation, inflammation and spasm of the lower gullet.

When the symptoms are typical, like those above, investigation is unnecessary.

When confirmation is required either a barium meal or endoscopy (painless examination with a flexible tube) is performed.

Some people with gastro-oesophageal reflux have a hiatus hernia but many people have reflux without hiatus hernias.

A hiatus hernia occurs when the upper portion of the stomach slips through the hole in the diaphragm (hiatus) into the chest. It is not dangerous and the vast majority of people with a hiatus hernia do not require an operation.

Gastro-oesophageal reflux is increased by

some foods (fats, pastry)
smoking
alcohol
very large meals
stooping or slumping in a chair
being overweight
tight clothing

These should therefore be avoided.

Raising the head of the bed by 10–15 cm often prevents reflux at night (extra pillows are of very little use).

Medical treatment with antacids, drugs to suppress acid secretion, e.g. Tagamet and Zantac, or other preparations such as Pyrogastrone, Gastro-cote and Gaviscon, is usually successful.

They may need to be used regularly for several months before relief is complete.

Like many forms of dyspepsia recurrence is common but surgery is only *very rarely* required.

An extremely rare complication is the formation of a narrowing of the gullet, which causes food to actually stick during swallowing. If this occurs contact your doctor who will arrange referral to hospital for additional treatment.

## INFORMATION FOR PATIENTS WITH PEPTIC ULCER

Peptic ulcers are either gastric (in the stomach) or duodenal.

The duodenum is the first part of the intestine into which the stomach empties.

Ulceration takes place when acid and other irritant substances produced in the stomach erode the lining of the stomach or duodenum.

Why this happens in some people and not others is unknown.

Hereditary factors play some part because ulcers tend to 'run in families'.

Other factors which probably predispose to ulcers are:

smoking,
excessive coffee,
aspirin and drugs used for arthritis.

Pain in the upper abdomen is the commonest symptom but others include heartburn and vomiting.

Diagnosis is confirmed by barium meal X-ray or endoscopy (painless examination of stomach and duodenum with a flexible tube).

Symptoms can usually be relieved by

regular antacids 2 hours after meals and before bedtime,
three normal meals per day (special diets are unnecessary),
stopping coffee, alcohol and smoking,
avoiding foods that consistently cause your pain.

Once the diagnosis has been confirmed your doctor will probably prescribe a 4–6 week course of Tagamet (cimetidine), Zantac (ranitidine), Gastrozepine (pirenzipine), Denol or sucralfate, to heal the ulcer.

Many ulcers remain healed for months or years and continuous treatment will not then be needed.

Unfortunately some ulcers rapidly recur and under these circumstances many doctors now advise continuous treatment for a year or more with a small daily dose of Tagamet or Zantac.

Nearly all ulcers recur at some time but with modern treatment they can be healed rapidly and for this reason surgery has become less popular.

Nevertheless, if recurrences are very frequent or if a complication such as bleeding occurs, an operation may be necessary.

## INFORMATION FOR PATIENTS WITH THE IRRITABLE BOWEL SYNDROME

In the past, many names have been given to this condition, e.g. mucous colitis, spastic colon, colonic dysfunction, nervous bowel, splenic and hepatic flexure syndromes.

It is very common – more than 10% of the UK population probably suffer from the disorder.

The exact cause is unknown, *but*

the basic abnormality is one of poor coordination of bowel muscle activity,

stress and emotional disturbance commonly bring on an attack,

in a few people gastroenteritis appears to be followed by an irritable bowel syndrome,

in others specific food items may be to blame although this is probably rare,

The commonest symptoms are

diffuse abdominal discomfort and sensation of distension, often made worse by food,

bouts of colicky pain, often before or after passing stool,

the need to open the bowels several times soon after rising in the morning,

pellet or thread shaped stools, sometimes coated with mucus,

constipation.

It is usual to perform a few routine blood tests, examination of the back passage and a barium enema to exclude other diseases.

*Avoid:*

(1)   emotional stress – if possible!
(2)   foods that bring on the symptoms

*For constipation,* cereals containing bran and wholemeal bread are helpful.

*For distension,* it may be necessary to reduce 'gas forming' foods and follow a low flatulence diet, or on some occasions a low fibre diet.

*Pain* can often be relieved by antispasmodic drugs from the general practitioner.

*Diarrhoea* is best relieved by small doses of loperamide (Imodium) or codeine phosphate.

*Tranquillizers* are sometimes useful when symptoms are very severe, and particularly when precipitated by unavoidable stresses.

The disorder is *not* related to:

ulcerative colitis,
Crohn's disease or
cancer.

It does *not* progress to more serious problems but often continues intermittently for several years.

## INFORMATION SHEET FOR PATIENTS WITH ULCERATIVE COLITIS

Ulcerative colitis is an inflammatory disease of the large intestine.

The exact cause is unknown.

It is *not* an infectious disease and other members of the family and friends are not at risk.

The principal symptoms are diarrhoea, and bleeding from the bowel.

A few patients also have inflammation of the eyes, skin or joints.

It tends to be a chronic disorder which may be subject to acute relapses over a period of many years.

Acute attacks are treated with steroids (usually prednisolone) either by tablets or enemas.

Occasionally severe attacks may require admission to hospital for additional treatment.

The number of relapses can be greatly reduced by regularly taking sulphasalazine (Salazopyrine) or 5-aminosalicylic acid which may be necessary for many years.

Most patients with colitis do not need special diets.

Follow-up at a hospital is usually advised but annual attendance is often all that is necessary.

In the majority of cases medical management is usually successful but a small minority who have:

extremely active disease, or
frequent relapses despite medication, or
general ill health over a long period, or
severe inflammation of eyes, skin or joints

may be advised to have the large intestine removed (colectomy).

Most patients with colitis live a normal life but adjustments may be necessary during serious relapses.

It is likely that the exact nature of ulcerative colitis will be discovered during the next few years, which could lead to the development of a complete cure for the disease.

*Mention of the increased risk of colorectal cancer is intentionally omitted* because it is not relevant to the patient's initial understanding of the disease and needs to be discussed only when the disorder has been present for more than 8 years.

## INFORMATION SHEET FOR PATIENTS WITH CROHN'S DISEASE

Crohn's disease is an inflammatory condition which affects either the large or small intestine, or both.

The exact cause is unknown.

It is *not* an infectious disease and other members of the family and friends are not at risk.

The principal symptoms are diarrhoea, abdominal pain and bleeding from the bowel.

A few patients also have inflammation of the eyes, skin or joints.

It tends to be a chronic disorder which may be subject to acute relapses over a period of many years.

Acute attacks are treated with steroids (usually prednisolone), either by tablets or enemas.

Occasionally severe attacks may require admission to hospital for additional treatment.

Crohn's disease often remits without treatment but a small amount of prednisolone is often needed to keep the disease under control. Salazopyrine, 5-aminosalicylic acid, or azathioprine are also used to prevent relapses and may be given for many years.

Most patients with Crohn's disease do not need special diets.

In many cases medical management is successful, but surgery may be needed in those who have:

extremely active disease, or
frequent relapses despite medication, or
severe inflammation of eyes, skin or joints, or
when inflammation has caused irreparable damage which cannot be relieved with drugs.

These may need resection of a part of the bowel.

# INFORMATION FOR PATIENTS WITH DIVERTICULAR DISEASE

Diverticula are small outpouchings that form in the large intestine. They are very common in those over 60 years of age.

The exact cause is unknown but patients with the disorder often have abnormal motility of the bowel.

In some cases the bowel wall becomes permanently thickened, which may result in recurrent constipation and pain in the lower abdomen.

A diverticulum may be the site of inflammation which gives rise to more severe pain and tenderness over the area involved. A mild fever often occurs in these circumstances.

Occasionally a diverticulum may bleed, which results in blood being passed from the back passage.

The diagnosis is confirmed by a barium enema X-ray examination.

If constipation is a major symptom increasing the fibre content of the diet – e.g. bran-containing cereals and wholemeal bread – may be helpful.

When pain is the main problem this can be relieved by antispasmodic and pain-relieving drugs from your doctor.

If inflammation is present antibiotics will be prescribed.

Whenever pain is severe you should immediately stop all solid food and take only fluids for a few days.

If the symptoms do not respond to this treatment admission to hospital is occasionally necessary. Only very rarely is an operation required.

Diverticular disease is in *no way* related to cancer.

## LOW RESIDUE DIET

This diet has been designed to minimize the amount of food residue (or roughage) to be excreted from your system.

Your aim should be to eat as normally as possible but of foods chosen from the list of 'Suitable Foods' below;

*In general avoid all fruits, vegetables and nuts, and any wholegrain cereal foods or those containing Bran.*

### Sample menu

#### Breakfast

Suitable cereal (see list below)
Strained fruit juice
Egg/bacon/fish (preferably not fried)
White bread or toast
Butter, jelly jam, honey, jelly marmalade
Tea, coffee.

#### Lunch

Clear soup, strained fruit juice
Meat, fish, egg, cheese dish
Potatoes, rice, spaghetti or white bread or rolls
Suitable vegetable, e.g. marrow
Suitable pudding, e.g. plain jelly, plain yogurt, plain cake or biscuits

#### Evening meal

As lunch

| Suitable foods | Unsuitable foods |
|---|---|
| **Bread**<br>White breads, rolls and scones, Energen rolls, Nimble, Slimcea | All brown or wholemeal breads, rolls and scones, matzos, crispbreads e.g. Ryvita |
| **Cereals**<br>Rice Crispies, Special-K, oatmeal porridge, white rice, macaroni, spaghetti | Bran cereals, shredded wheat, puffed wheat, cornflakes, Weetabix, wholemeal flour and wholewheat pasta |
| **Biscuits** (in moderation)<br>Smooth types e.g. Rich Tea, shortcake, custard creams | Digestive, oatcakes, crispbread e.g. Ryvita, wholewheat biscuits, any containing fruit or nuts including coconut |
| **Cakes, pudding & sweets**<br>Plain sponge, Yorkshire pudding, pancakes, Madeira cake, meringues, eclairs, baked or boiled custards, junket, plain yoghurt, ice cream, plain jellies, rice pudding, pastry (made with white flour). | Cakes or puddings containing wholemeal flour or cereals. Any containing dried or fresh fruit, dates, nuts |
| **Preserves**<br>Shredless marmalade, jelly jams, honey, lemon curd, golden syrup | Jams containing pips or skins |
| **Fruits** (in moderation)<br>Peeled de-seeded grapes, canned grapefruit segments, canned mandarin oranges, fresh or canned lychees, melon flesh, strained fruit juices except prune juice | All other fruits, fresh, canned, frozen or dried<br>All nuts<br>Prune juice |
| **Vetetables** (in moderation)<br>Potatoes – boiled , mashed, new, marrow, courgettes – peeled and boiled, cucumber – peeled, Lettuce – tender no stalks, canned tomatoes – no skins or pips | All other vegetables |

| Suitable foods | Unsuitable foods |
| --- | --- |
| *Meat* | |
| All tender meats, fresh or frozen (preferably not fried) | Salt or cured meats, sausages |
| *Eggs* | |
| Preferably not fried | |
| *Cheeses* | |
| All in moderation | |
| *Fish* | |
| All, preferably not fried | |
| *Miscellaneous* | |
| Sugar, boiled sweets, peppermints, other sweets in moderation | Cocoa, liquorice sweets, fruit or nut confectionery, marzipan. |
| Clear soups, Oxo, Bovril, Marmite | All chutneys and pickles |
| Salt, pepper, vinegar, salad cream, mayonnaise | Yeast tablets |
| Ribena, strained fruit squash, lime cordial, fizzy drinks | |

## DIET FOR RELIEF OF FLATULENCE

Flatulence is caused by the accumulation of gas in the stomach and intestines. Of this gas, more than half is air which is swallowed during eating and drinking – and even talking; the rest is formed by the action of the bacteria in the gut on food residues. About 500 ml of this mixture of gases is passed every day as a *normal* biological function.

Flatulence is thus reduced by minimizing the amount or air swallowed and avoiding certain foods.

*A.  To reduce the amount of air swallowed:*

(1)  Set aside enough time for a meal – eat slowly and relax for a time afterwards

(2)  Do not 'gulp' food or drink

(3)  Avoid very hot or very cold foods which are swallowed quickly

(4)  Avoid fizzy drinks

*B.  The following foods contain certain sugars which are not digested* and can cause gas formation in the bowel:

(1)  Peas, beans (baked beans, haricot, butter beans etc.) lentils and other pulses

(2)  Certain root vegetables – parsnips, Jerusalem artichokes, turnips, onions

(3)  Some nuts if eaten in large quantities, e.g. chestnuts

(4)  Raw cabbage, e.g. in coleslaw

(5)  Molasses

(6)  Cutting down on sugar and sweet foods and drinks – e.g. biscuits, sweets, lemonade and fruit squashes, fruit tinned in heavy syrup – can bring relief

(7)  In rare cases consumption of large amounts of milk and milk products causes wind

*C.  Avoid constipation* by increasing *gradually* the amount of cereal fibre in your diet. The following foods will help:

(1)  Wholemeal bread or bread with added bran, e.g. Hi-Bran

(2)  Wholemeal flour in cakes and crumbles, pastries and biscuits etc

(3) Wholewheat cereals – Weetabix, Shredded Wheat, Puffed Wheat; bran cereals – All-Bran, farmhouse bran, branflakes etc.

(4) Unprocessed bran (if needed) should also be introduced gradually. Start with 1 dessertspoon and increase to 2 – 3 tablespoons daily; mix with yogurt or sprinkle over any suitable food such as cereal, porridge, stewed fruit.

(5) Be sure to take plenty of fluids – at least 10–12 cups a day

D. *If your intake of vegetables has been reduced*, it is important to take an extra source of vitamin C every day. This can be obtained from:

(1) citrus fruits – oranges, grapefruits, tangerines etc

(2) unsweetened fruit juice – orange or grapefruit

(3) rosehip syrup

## HIGH FIBRE DIET

### Introduction

Fibre is a complex mixture of plant substances which we do not digest or absorb. However, it is very necessary for the proper working of the intestine. It acts by passing unchanged through the intestine where it absorbs water, increases the bulk of undigested food and helps muscles in their important function of pushing the food residue along the intestines, so preventing constipation and straining.

Many people's diet in this country is lacking in fibre. This is because they eat little plant food and the plant food they do eat has been processed in such a way as to remove and destroy the fibre – e.g. white flour, where the fibre-rich outer layers have been removed in the milling process.

### High fibre foods

There are three main food sources of dietary fibre:

(1)  *Bran and wholegrain cereals*. These are a more concentrated source of fibre. When following a high fibre diet, change to using wholegrain cereals such as wholemeal bread, wholemeal flour, brown rice and wholewheat breakfast cereals or bran breakfast cereal.

 Fibre may be increased further if necessary by adding unprocessed bran to the diet. Bran can be bought at most health food stores, supermarkets and chemists.

(2)  *Fruit, vegetables and nuts*. Fibre from these foods is higher in the skin and peel. When following a high fibre diet always, where possible, eat the skin and peel and try to eat the food raw or only lightly cooked, as cooking breaks down the fibre.

(3)  *Pulses*. Try to include these in your diet daily. Use them in soups, stews and salads or as a vegetable. Pulses are: peas, lentils, baked beans and beans such as butter, red kidney, haricot, black eye, aduke, crab eye, mung and soya.

### Guidelines for using bran

When starting to use unprocessed bran you may experience some flatulence or wind at first, but this will only be temporary – do not stop taking bran because of it.

You will find that the amount of bran necessary will depend on the quantity of fibre in the rest of your diet. Once you have found the correct dose of bran for yourself, continue to take this indefinitely unless directed otherwise by your doctor or dietitian.

It is better when taking bran for the first time to introduce it slowly into your diet, e.g.

(1)  One heaped teaspoon bran three times daily before meals or with the first course

(2)  Increase the dose after 1 week by one heaped teaspoon bran

(3)  Continue to increase the dose by one heaped teaspon each week until the motions are of a soft consistency and passed without effort

## Some ways of taking bran

(1)  Dry but washed down with a glass of water, milk, fruit juice or other liquid

(2)  Sprinkle on any other foods

(3)  Moisten bran with a small amount of boiling water and then add to food or drink

(4)  Mixed with breakfast cereals

(5)  Add to homemade cakes, bread, biscuits and pastry etc

(6)  Add to soups, sauces, stews, gravies, custard etc.

Ensure that an adequate fluid intake is taken daily – at least 10 cups (or 8 mugs) in the form of tea, coffee, water, fruit juice etc.

## Foods with high fibre content

### Breakfast cereals

All-Bran, Bran Buds, Weetabix, Shredded Wheat, oats, Alpen, muesli

### Flour

Wholewheat or whole rye of 100% extraction

### Bread

Any made from wholewheat or whole rye flour of 100% extraction

## Rice and pasta

Use brown rice or add bran to white rice; wholewheat macaroni or spaghetti

## Cakes and biscuits

Made with wholewheat flour, oatmeal or rolled oats, dried fruit and nuts. Digestive, Hi Bran or bran biscuits. Wholegrain crispbreads, e.g. Ryvita

## Fruit

All kinds in generous amounts and raw with the skins when possible

## Vegetables and pulses

All kinds in generous amounts – as much raw as possible. Potatoes should be boiled or baked in their skins. Peas, lentils and dried beans – e.g. butter beans, black eye beans

## Nuts

All kinds

## Suggested meal patterns

### Breakfast

Porridge or high fibre cereal
Egg, bacon, fish – if desired
Bread made with 100% wholewheat flour
Butter or margarine
Coarse marmalade
Tea or Coffee or fruit juice

### Mid-morning

Tea or coffee or milk or fruit juice
Digestive or bran biscuits or fresh fruit, if desired

### Lunch/evening meal

Serving of homemade vegetable soup
Serving of meat/chicken/fish/egg/cheese

Potatoes cooked in their skins or brown rice
*or* wholemeal bread/wholemeal pasta
Large helping of lightly cooked vegetables/salad
Fresh or stewed fruit or pudding made with fruit and nuts
Tea or coffee or fruit juice

### Mid-afternoon

Tea or coffee/milk/fruit juice
Digestive or bran biscuits or wholewheat bread

### Suppliers of wholemeal bread – 100% extraction

Health food stores
Some baker's shops and supermarkets (e.g. Sainsbury's, Marks and Spencer)

*Always ask for Allinson's bread or equivalent*

### Suppliers of Bran

Health food stores
Chemists, e.g. Boots, and some supermarkets.

Ask for: Allinson's Natural Bran Plus or Prewett's Natural Unprocessed Bran

# Bibliography

*Oesophageal disease*

Truelove, S. C. and Ritchie, J. A. (1976).(eds.) *Topics in Gastroenterology 4*. (Oxford: Blackwell Scientific)
Atkinson, M. (1976). (ed). Disorders of oesophageal motility. *Clin. Gastroenterol.,* **5** (1).

*Peptic ulcer*

Truelove, S. C. and Jewell, D. P. (1973). (eds.) *Topics in Gastroenterology, 1*. (Oxford: Blackwell Scientific)
Truelove, S. C. and Willoughby, C. P. (1979). (eds.) *Topics in Gastroenterology, 7*. (Oxford: Blackwell Scientific)
Truelove, S. C. and Heyworth, M. F. (1978). (eds.) *Topics in Gastroenterology, 6*. (Oxford: Blackwell Scientific)
Gear, M. W. L. (1983). Proximal gastric vagotomy versus long term maintenance treatment with cimetidine for chronic duodenal ulcer; a prospective randomized trial. *Br. Med. J.,* **286**, 98–9.
Lancaster Smith, M. J. (1983). *Peptic Ulcer,* Seminar. (London: Update Books)
Lancaster Smith, M. J. (1984). *Peptic Ulcer.* Seminar. (London: Update Publications)

*Gastrointestinal haemorrhage*

Torsoli, A. (ed.) (1981). Gastrointestinal emergencies. *Clin. Gastroenterol.* **10** (1)

Truelove, S. C. and Goodman, M. J. (1975). (eds.) *Topics in Gastroenterology, 3.* (Oxford: Blackwell Scientific)

*Irritable bowel syndrome*

Truelove, S. C. and Jewell, D. P. (1973). (eds.) *Topics in Gastroenterology, 1.* (Oxford: Blackwell Scientific)

Almy, T. P. and Fielding, J. F. (eds.) (1977). The G.I. tract in stress and psychological disorder. *Clin. Gastroenterol.,* **6** (3)

*Inflammatory bowel disease*

Truelove, S. C. and Jewell, D. P. (1973). (eds.) *Topics in Gastroenterology 1,* (Oxford: Blackwell Scientific)

Truelove, S. C. and Kennedy, H. J. (1973). (eds.) *Topics in Gastroenterology 8.* (Oxford: Blackwell Scientific)

*Coeliac disease*

Truelove, S. C. and Ritchie, J. A. (1976). (eds.) *Topics in Gastroenterology, 4.* (Oxford: Blackwell Scientific)

Asquith, P. (ed.) (1979). *Immunology of the Gastrointestinal Tract.* (Edinburgh and London: Churchill Livingstone)

*Liver and bilary system – general*

Wright, R., Alberti, K. G. M. M., Karvan, S. and Millward-Sailler, G. H. (eds.) (1979). *Liver and Biliary Disease.* (Philadelphia: Saunders)

Sherlock, S. (1981). *Disease of the Liver and Biliary System.* 6th Edn. (Oxford: Blackwell Scientific)

*Hepatitis*

Truelove, S. C. and Goodman, M. J. (1975). (eds.) *Topics in Gastroenterology, 3.* (Oxford: Blackwell Scientific)

Truelove, S. C. and Ritchie, J. A. (1976). (eds.) *Topics in Gastroenterology, 4.* (Oxford: Blackwell Scientific)

Truelove, S. C. and Heyworth, M. F. (1978). (eds.) *Topics in Gastroenterology, 6.* (Oxford: Blackwell Scientific)

Weller I. (1984). Viral hepatitis. *Br. Med. J.* **288**, 47–9

*Drugs and the liver*

Truelove, S. C. and Lee, E. (1977). (eds.) *Topics in Gastroenterology, 5.* (Oxford: Blackwell Scientific)


*Gastrointestinal cancer*

Sherlock, P. Zamcheck, N. (eds.) (1976). Cancer of the G.I. tract. *Clin. Gastroenterol.*, **5** (3)

Lallemand, R. C., Vakil, P. A., Pearson, P. and Box, V. (1984). Screening for asymptomatic bowel cancer in general practice. *Br. Med. J.*, **288**, 31–3


*Gastroenteritis*

Lambert, H. P. (ed.) (1979). Infections of the G.I. tract. *Clin. Gastroenterol.*, **8** (3)

Prescribing for Acute Diarrhoea. *Drug Ther. Bull.* (1983), **21,** 101–4


*The acute abdomen*

Torsoli, A. (ed.) (1981). Gastrointestinal emergencies. *Clin. Gastroenterol.*, **10** (1)


*Miscellaneous*

Alexander Williams, J. (1983). Causes and management of anal irritation. *Br. Med. J.*, **287**, 1528

# Index

achalasia
  and carcinoma   16
  cardiomyotomy   15, 16
  causes   14
  management   15, 16
  symptoms   15
acid perfusion test   5
Addison's disease   20
adverse drug reactions
  antacids   31
  anticholinergic drugs   34
  carbenoxolone   33
  cimetidine   30
  laxatives   136, 137
aerophagy
  belching   143
  pain   79
alcohol
  abuse
    bowel function   95
    jaundice   146–8
    peptic ulcer   41
    vomiting   22, 23
  withdrawal management   163
alcoholic liver disease   161–3
  categories   161
  and consumption   161, 162
  diagnosis   161
  patient advice   161, 162
  prognosis   163
  survival rates   162, 163
alkaline phosphatase in jaundice   149

5–aminosalicylic acid   120
anaemia   8, 104
  diarrhoea   96
  folate deficiency   104
  gastrectomy   50, 51, 54, 55
anal fissure   62
anal irritation
  causes   144
  management   144
angiodysplasia   64
anorexia, features   141
anorexia nervosa   141
  features and management   21, 23
antacids, buffering capacities   31, 32
antibiotic-induced diarrhoea   90
antireticulum antibody   107
aortic aneurysm, pain in ruptured   67, 72, 73
appendicitis, features of pain   69
arthritis in inflammatory bowel
    disease   126
ascitis   158
  recurrence and treatment   159
aspirin in peptic ulcer bleeding   39, 41

bad breath   142
  causes and significance   143
barium enema
  Crohn's disease   124
  double contrast   62, 63, 99, 100
barium meal
  dyspepsia   81

gastro-oesophageal reflux  4
  peptic ulcer  29
bile salt breath test  109, 110
biliary colic  66
  features of pain  71
bilirubin, serum levels in jaundice  149
biopsy
  liver in jaundice  150, 151
  small bowel diagnosis  106, 108
bismuth in peptic ulcer  32, 33
bowel action frequency  133
bowel colic  66
bowel ischaemia, pain  73
bran
  in constipation  134
  guidelines for use  178, 179
  suppliers  181
bulimia nervosa  141
  features and management  21, 22

*Campylobacter* spp., enteritis features  86
candidiasis  16
carbenoxolone in peptic ulcer  33
carcinoid syndrome, diarrhoea
  features  98, 99
carcinoma *see also individual organs*
  postcricoid  10
cardiomyotomy  15, 16
cholangiography in jaundice  151, 152
cholecystitis, pain features  71
cholestasis in jaundice  155
cimetidine in peptic ulcer  30, 31
cirrhosis
  alcoholic  161
  causes  158
  decompensated  158, 159
  and jaundice  147, 155
  mental deterioration  161
*Clostridium difficile,* pseudomembranous
    colitis  91
clubbing, finger nail  105
coeliac disease  99, 103
  associated conditions  108
  biopsy  106, 108
  gluten role and diet  108
colonoscopy, chronic diarrhoea  100
colorectal cancer
  constipation  137, 139
  diagnosis  96
  pain  79, 82
  sigmoidoscopy  139
  ulcerative colitis  121, 122
constipation
  alternating diarrhoea  138
  causes  137, 138
  definition  133

management  134, 135
  prophylaxis  135
Crohn's disease
  bleeding  63
  diarrhoea  95
  investigation  81
  malabsorption  103
  pain  78
  rectum  97
  abscesses  123, 124
  animal investigations  126
  bleeding  63
  cancer risk  126
  diagnostic techniques  124
  diarrhoea  95
  immune response  123
  incidence, UK  122
  investigation  81
  malabsorption  103
  management  124, 171
    long-term  125
  pain  78
  patient information  170, 171
  prophylactic drugs  125
  rectum  97
  surgery incidence  125, 171
  symptoms  123
defaecation problems  133–9; *see also*
    constipation
  reflex  133
dermatitis herpetiformis  105, 109
dermatomyositis  16
descending perineum syndrome  138
diabetes mellitus and diarrhoea  98
diaphragm, pinchcock action  1
diarrhoea
  acute, infective *see* gastroenteritis
  chronic  93–100
  definition  93
  drug-induced  90, 91, 95
  duration  93
  examination  95, 96
  investigations  96–9
  management of infectious  89, 90
  pain  67
  parasites  89
  peptic ulcer surgery  49, 52
  radiological findings  99, 100
  salmonella  84, 85
  sigmoidoscopy  96, 97
  spurious in elderly  94, 95
  travellers', causes  87–9
diet
  diverticulitis  131
  fibre  134
  gluten-free  108

hepatitis   152
high-fibre   176–80
high residue   174, 175
irritable bowel syndrome   114
low flatulence   144, 176, 177
low residue foods   173–5
peptic ulcer   26, 29, 37
vitamin C   177
diffuse oesophageal spasm   15
diverticular disease   63
  bowel obstruction   130
  diet   129
  diffuse and sigmoid   129
  incidence and age   129
  management   130, 131
  pain   79, 131
  patient information   172
  perforation   130
diverticulitis
  definition and features   130
  pain features   70
  surgery   131
  treatment, acute   131
  vaginal fistulae   130
drugs
  diarrhoea   90, 91, 95
  hepatitis   156
  –induced hepatic dysfunction   157
  jaundice   148
dumping   49
  mechanisms and peptic ulcer   53, 54
duodenal ulcer
  pain features   76
  surgery   45–51
  diarrhoea   49
  dumping   49
  gastrectomy   50
  nutritional effects   50, 51
  patient selection   45–7
  proximal gastric vagotomy   49
  recurrence, incidence   47
  techniques   46, 48–50
  techniques and mortality   47
  vagotomy and antrectomy   48
  vagotomy and pyloroplasty   48
dysentery, features of shigella   85
dyspepsia
  pain features   76, 80
  stress   80
dysphagia
  conditions causing   16
  cortical and age   11
  definition   9
  neuromuscular, causes   10, 11
  oesophageal, causes   12–16
  pharyngeal, causes   9–12

encephalopathy, hepatic
  causes   159, 160
  chronic, treatment   160
  hospital admission   160
  management objectives   159
endoscopic retrograde
    cholangiopancreatography
    (ERCP)   152, 153
endoscopy
  benign peptic stricture   13
  gastro-oesophageal reflux   5
  gut lesion   60
  peptic ulcer   60
Entamoeba histolytica
  features of infection   88
  travellers' diarrhoea   88
  treatment   89
Escherichia coli
  small bowel pathogenicity   84
  travellers' diarrhoea   87

faecal fat, excretion   107, 108
faecal impaction   134
fibre see also diet
  suggested meals   180, 181
  use in cooking   180
folate deficiency   55

gallbladder disease
  investigations   82
  pain features   71, 80
gas in alimentary tract   143, 144
  foods causing   144, 176
gastrectomy
  Billroth   48, 52
  duodenal ulcer   48, 50
  gastric ulcer   51, 52
  Polya   48, 54
gastric acid production, drugs reducing   6,
    29, 30
  see also cimetidine, ranitidine
gastric cancer   57, 58
  pain features   76, 77
gastric pressure   5, 6
gastric surgery
  heartburn   7
  malabsorption   102, 103
gastric ulcer
  pain features   76
  surgery   51–5
    anaemia   54, 55
    diarrhoea   52
    dumping mechanisms   53, 54
    operations and mortality   51, 52
    osteomalacia   55
    patient selection   51

recurrence 52
gastritis pain 79
gastroenteritis
  bacteria causing 84–7
  causes and pain features 70
  features 80
  toxin-induced 83, 84
gastrointestinal absorption processes 101,
    102; *see also* malabsorption
gastrointestinal haemorrhage 57–64; *see
    also* rectal
  causes 41, 59, 60
  chronic, causes 60, 61
  hypovolaemia 61
  types 57
  upper acute, causes 57, 58
    blood loss 59
    gut lesion 60
    mortality and age 57, 58
    severity assessment 58, 59
gastrojejunostomy 46
gastro-oesophageal reflux
  aspiration 3
  factors increasing 166
  investigations 4, 5
  management 3–5, 7
  measurement 5
  mechanisms controlling 1, 2
  motor activity control 2
  patient information 165, 166
  predisposing conditions 7, 8
  referral rate 1
  surgery, indications 8
  symptoms 2, 3
  treatment 5–7
*Giardia lamblia* 97
  Leningrad 88
  travellers diarrhoea 87, 88
Gilbert's disease 146
globus syndrome 12, 17

haematemesis 40, 58
  coffee grounds 58
  recurrence 60
haemochromatosis 158
haemorrhoids, treatment of bleeding 62
heartburn
  causes 2
  drugs contraindicated 7
  gastro-oesophageal reflux 2, 3, 165
  peptic ulcer 28
  pregnancy 7
Henoch–Schönlein purpura 73
hepatic carcinoma 147
hepatitis
  alcohol and type A 154

chronic 155
chronic active 156, 157
  management 156, 157
chronic persistent 155, 156
drug-induced 156, 157
fulminant 155
lupoid 157
prednisolone 157
viral
  complications 154
  non-A, non-B 154, 156
  persistence 156
  type A, features and diagnosis 152,
    154
  type B, prevention 154, 156
hepatoma and jaundice 155
hepatomegaly 149
hiatus hernia 165
  sliding 4
Hirschsprung's disease 138
hookworm 61

impotence 160
inflammatory bowel disease *see also*
    Crohn's, ulcerative colitis
  childhood 127
  complications 126, 127
  defaecation 94
  pregnancy 127
intestinal obstruction 20
  causes 72
  pain features 71, 72
intra-abdominal arterial grafts 61
intrinsic factor 10
irritable bowel syndrome 111–15, 134
  constipation 134, 138
  diarrhoea 93, 94, 96, 113, 138, 168
  diet 114, 168
  drug use 114, 115, 169
  eating role 111
  gas 144
  incomplete bowel emptying 139
  management 113
  pain, features 76–8, 112
  prevalence 111, 168
  relapsing 115
  stress role 113, 114
  symptoms 168

jaundice
  cholestatic, causes 146, 147
  classification 145
  clinical features 147–9
  definition 145
  drugs inducing 148
  haemolytic 146

hepatocellular, causes   146, 147
hyperbilirubinaemia   145, 146
non-haemolytic   146
investigations   149–53
scheme   153
serum enzymes   149, 150

laparoscopy in jaundice   151
laxatives   134, 135
types and problems   136, 137
laxative abuse
bowel re-education   136
colonic cancer   135
patient features   99, 135
libido loss   160
liquorice, deglycyrrhizinized in peptic
ulcer   33
liver disorders in inflammatory bowel
disease   127
lump in the throat   117

malabsorption syndrome   101–10
anaemia   110
biopsy   106
causes   101–3
diarrhoea   103
investigations   106–8
mucosal disease   101
nutritional deficiency   104, 105
radiology   107
signs   103-6
small intestine colonization   102, 103,
109, 110
small intestine resection   101
vitamin $B_{12}$ 110
melaena   3
assessment   59
peptic ulcer   40
Menière's disease, vomiting   22
mesenteric adenitis, pain   69, 70
mesenteric angina, pain   78
metoclopramide   5
metronidazole and alcohol   88
migraine, vomiting   22
mortality
gastrointestinal haemorrhage   58
peptic ulcer surgery   47, 51, 52
myocardial infarction   68, 73

nausea   19
Norwalk agent   87

oesophageal carcinoma
achalasia   16
diagnosis   14
prognosis   14

treatment   14
types   13
oesophageal sphincter, competence and
reflux   5
oesophageal stricture, benign and
malignant   17
oesophagitis   4, 17, 58, 143
osteomalacia   105
peptic ulcer surgery   51, 54
treatment   160
oxyphenisatin   137

pain
acute abdominal   65–73 see also
individual conditions
causes and features   69–74
examination   68, 69
features   67, 68
inflammatory   68
sites and onset   65–7
chronic abdominal   75–82
causes and features   77–80
features   75
hepatic   80
management   81, 82
musculoskeletal   80
postprandial   75–7, 112
renal   80
jaundice   147
pancreatic carcinoma   146
pain   78
pancreatitis
investigations   82
malabsorption   70, 78, 103, 109
tests   109
pain, features   70, 78
peptic disease, vomiting   22, 23
peptic stricture
benign, management   12, 13
dilatation   11
peptic ulcer
aetiological factors   26, 27, 167
antacids   31, 32
bismuth   32, 33
bleeding, incidence   38, 58
aspirin role   39, 41
blood group   39
severity   40
site   41
complicated   39–44
conditions confused   27
diagnosis   39
drug treatment   29–34
duodenal and gastric   25
$H_2$-antagonists   29–31, 167
healing and recurrence   34, 37

incidence, UK   25
long-term care   36, 38
management   28, 29
mortality   39
mucus role   26
pain   77
   management   81, 82
pathogenic mechanisms   25, 26
patient information   167
penetration   42, 43
perforation, occurrence   41
   pain and shock   42, 71
   reduction   42
prognosis   36, 37
prophylaxis   35
referral   38
relapse rate   35, 36, 167
   and surgery   47, 48, 52
severity assessment   36
surgery   45–55; *see also* duodenal *and*
      gastric
   incidence   37
   operations   46, 48–50
symptoms   28
uncomplicated   25–38
percutaneous transhepatic cholangiography
      in jaundice   152, 153
pericarditis   73
peristalsis, secondary   1
peritonitis   67
pharyngeal pouch, diagnosis and
   management   9, 10
pharyngo-oesophageal web   10
pirenzepine in peptic ulcer   34
polyposis
   large intestine   62, 63
   small intestine   61
polyps, large bowel   62, 63
prednisolone in hepatitis   157
pregnancy
   anorexia   141
   constipation   134
   ectopic, pain   72
   nausea and vomiting   20, 141
proctalgia fugax   139
prostaglandins in peptic ulcer   34
protein-losing enteropathy   105
pseudomembranous colitis
   features and drugs   90
   toxins   91
pyelonephritis, pain features   73
pyloric stenosis   43, 44
   causes   20
   diagnosis   43
   peptic ulcer   43
   treatment   43, 44

vomiting   43
pyloroplasty   46
pyrogastrone and ulcers   6

radio-isotope scanning, cirrhosis   151
ranitidine in peptic ulcer   31
rectal carcinoma   63
   incomplete emptying sensation   138
rectal examination   62, 68
   blood   96
rectal haemorrhage   61–4, 67
   causes   62–4
   colonic ischaemia   64
   infections   63
   investigations   62
   massive, causes   64
rectum, solitary ulcer   138, 139
renal colic   66
   features   73, 80

*Salmonella typhimurium*   84
salpingitis, pain features   72
Schatzski's ring   13
Schilling test   110
scleroderma   7, 16
*Shigella* spp. dysentery, management   85
sigmoidoscopy   62, 63
   chronic diarrhoea   96, 97
   Crohn's disease   124
   ulcerative colitis   118
small bowel stagnation and bacteria   102,
      103
smoking and gastric ulcer   26, 37
steatorrhoea   94
   malabsorption   103
stool
   description of normal   93
   microbiology   97
sucralfate, antipepsin   33
sulphasalazine in ulcerative colitis   119,
      120

telangiectasia   60
thyrotoxicosis, diarrhoea   98
tongue, features of abnormal   142
toxins and diarrhoea   83, 84, 91
trimipramine in peptic ulcer   34
tropical sprue   89

ulcerative colitis (proctocolitis)
   animal investigations   122
   bleeding   63
   causes   117
   colectomy   120
   colonic cancer risk   121, 122, 170
   diagnosis   118

diarrhoea   118
management   119, 170
  long-term   121
  mild disease   119, 120
  severe   120
  steroid use   120
patient information   170
prevalence, UK   117
severity and features   118
ulcers, buccal   142
ultrasound, role in jaundice   151

vagotomy   46–9
virus *see also* hepatitis
  diarrhoea   87
  gastric ulcer   27
vitamin $B_{12}$ malabsorption   110
vomiting
  acute, causes   19
  and diarrhoea   19

episodic   20–3
metabolic disease   20
peptic ulcer   28
  surgery   54
persistent, causes   19, 20
psychogenic   21

weight loss   104
  diarrhoea   95
  gastrectomy   51
Wilson's disease   156–8
  and copper   158

xylose absorption test   107

*Yersinia* spp. and Crohn's disease   122, 123
*Yersinia enterocolitica*, diarrhoea features   86, 87